ENHANCING YOUR
ENDOCANNABINOID SYSTEM

JUSTIN KANDER, MS

TABLE OF CONTENTS

I. INTRODUCTION

Health is the most important asset you have. Without health, everything else in life becomes meaningless. Some people can live well with minor health problems, while others are confined to their homes because of debilitating disease. Regardless of severity, everyone seeks a life without medical issues. When in a perfectly healthy state, you are free to live life to the fullest.

Of course, health is more than just the absence of disease. There are many people who are not formally diagnosed with a condition, but still exhibit signs of imperfect health. General anxiety, lethargy, lack of energy, mental fog, and a disconnected mindset plague many otherwise healthy people. Alleviating these impediments is critical to optimal living and society's progress, but modern medicine has little to offer. Even for major diseases, traditional pharmaceutical options often only help manage symptoms and delay disease progression. While pharmaceuticals certainly help millions of people, better options are direly needed for so many others.

The endocannabinoid system (ECS) may be the ideal pharmacological target for restoring overall health. This chemical messaging system is responsible for maintaining homeostasis, or stable balance, in all vertebrates. Theoretically, when an organism is in homeostasis, there should be an absence of disease. Essentially by definition, if an organism is not in perfect homeostasis, there will be some level of disease.

How disease manifests is dependent on a variety of genetic and environmental factors, but most conditions involve some dysfunction of the ECS.

Given the above fact, it makes sense that enhancing the ECS, as well as using medicines that work through it, could potentially treat a wide variety of diseases. If homeostasis can be restored, then diseases should be better managed or potentially eliminated. While the nature of ECS dysfunction or deficiency varies between diseases, and thus may require different approaches, the predominant goal of restoring normal function is always the same.

At its heart, the ECS is all about communication. When cells communicate efficiently, everything works as it should. The body will be disease-free, and the mind will be clear and focused. Every human should work to optimize their health as a means of preventing disease and living well. By targeting the ECS, there is a clear map to achieving great health.

The ECS can be enhanced through a variety of non-cannabis and cannabis-based techniques. Cannabis is especially powerful because its plant cannabinoids (phytocannabinoids) are functionally similar to the endogenous cannabinoids (endocannabinoids) used by the ECS. Phytocannabinoids mimic the actions of endocannabinoids, such as activating specific cannabinoid receptors. In cases where endocannabinoids are not enough to maintain homeostasis, phytocannabinoids appear to act as a direct support system. While extracts from cannabis are undoubtedly very valuable, it is critical to embrace other enhancement measures to facilitate the body's optimal use of phytocannabinoids.

The following section discusses the basics of the ECS, its role as a protective network, and the research showing how it is connected to most diseases imaginable. It is not completely necessary to understand all these scientific details, and many people may prefer to skip to the ECS enhancement section. For convenience, the Conclusion section summarizes the most important advice, although it lacks the explanations of preceding sections. In any case, it is always good to know more about how something works, and seeing the incredible research behind the ECS provides confidence that enhancing it is worthwhile.

II. COMPONENTS OF THE ENDOCANNABINOID SYSTEM

The endocannabinoid system is a chemical messaging system in vertebrates that consists of endocannabinoids, cannabinoid receptors, and enzymes that synthesize and degrade the endocannabinoids, along with other regulatory components (Lu & Mackie, 2021). These endogenous compounds produced within the body have similar chemical structures to the external phytocannabinoids in the cannabis plant. The purpose of this system is to maintain homeostasis, which fundamentally is the maintenance of internal characteristics in the presence of external chances. Practically, this consists of regulating stable energy and hormone levels, neurotransmitter concentrations, temperature, and more.

The two primary endocannabinoids include N-arachidonoyl ethanolamine (anandamide) and 2-arachidonoyl glycerol (2-AG) (McPartland, 2008). Endocannabinoids are synthesized from essential fatty acids, including Omega-6 and Omega-3 fatty acids like arachidonic acid and eicosapentaenoic acid (EPA) respectively. Anandamide is mostly derived from N-arachidonoyl phosphatidyl ethanol via multiple pathways and degraded by fatty acid amide hydrolase (FAAH) (Lu & Mackie, 2016). 2-AG is generated mostly from arachidonoyl-containing phosphatidyl inositol bis-phosphate by the enzyme diacylglycerol lipase, and is degraded by monoacylglycerol lipase (MAGL).

There are three other known endocannabinoids and one additional compound that may be an endocannabinoid.

These include 2-arachidonoyl glycerol ether (2-AGE), O-arachidonoyl ethanolamine (also known as virodhamine), and N-arachidonoyl dopamine (Mannekote Thippaiah et al., 2021). Lysophosphatidylinositol may be the sixth endocannabinoid based on its interaction with a novel cannabinoid receptor (Piñeiro & Falasca, 2012). Other endocannabinoid-like compounds and analogs exist, but currently are not officially classified as endocannabinoids.

C. Endogenous cannabinoids (eicosanoids)

Anandamide (AEA)		$CB_1 \gg CB_2$ agonist TRPV$_1$ agonist	Mechoulam et al., 1995 Khanolkar et al., 1996 Schowalter et al., 1996 Felder et al., 1995 Zygmunt et al., 1999
2-Arachidonoyl glycerol (2-AG)		$CB_1 \approx CB_2$ agonist	Mechoulam et al., 1995 Ben-Shabat et al., 1998
2-Arachidonoyl glycerol ether		$CB_1 \gg CB_2$ agonist	Hanus et al., 2001
O-Arachidonoyl ethanolamine (virodhamine)		$CB_1 \gg CB_2$ agonist	Porter et al., 2002
N-Arachidonoyl dopamine		$CB_1 \gg CB_2$ agonist TRPV$_1$ agonist	Bisogno et al., 2000 Huang et al., 2002

(Pacher et al., 2006)

Cannabinoid receptors are the next fundamental part of the ECS. They are known as G protein-coupled receptors (GPCRs) because G (guanine nucleotide-binding) proteins are attached to them (Eglen et al., 2007).

Ligands are chemicals which activate receptors. When a receptor is stimulated by a ligand, the G protein detaches from the receptor and attaches to another compound, which induces a biological response by initiating a signaling cascade (McPartland, 2008). These cascades, or biochemical pathways, involve a series of second messengers which amplify the signal produced by the ligand, and subsequently produce one of a variety of cellular responses.

GPCRs have different subtypes, such as G_o, G_i, and G_s. These subtypes indicate what the G protein will couple to after receptor activation, such as ion channels or enzymes (McPartland, 2008). The cannabinoid receptors couple primarily to the G_i and G_o subtypes, meaning they inhibit adenylate cyclase (a key regulatory enzyme throughout nearly all cells) and activate ion channels respectively (Zou & Kumar, 2018).

The most prominent cannabinoid receptors are CB_1 and CB_2. CB_1 is the most abundant receptor in the mammalian brain; it is also found throughout the body in much lower concentrations (Chiarlone et al., 2014). CB_1 activation conveys the psychoactive effect of cannabis. Distribution of CB_1 is not uniform; the highest concentrations are in the basal ganglia, hippocampus, cerebral cortex, cerebellum, and amygdaloid nucleus. There are virtually no receptors in the brainstem, which controls breathing. This layout explains why THC and other activators of CB_1 receptors affect memory, emotion, cognition, motor function, and pain (McPartland, 2008). Also, the lack of cannabinoid receptors in the brainstem accounts for why overdosing on cannabis cannot cause death. However, the brainstem is replete with opioid receptors, which is why opioid drugs have the potential to stop respiration.

CB_2 is distributed primarily in cells throughout the immune and hematopoietic systems, meaning the receptors are found on white blood cells and tissues in the spleen, lymph nodes, bone marrow, and tonsils (Pacher et al., 2006). In lesser quantities, they are distributed throughout the brain, pancreas, and liver. Activation of this receptor can induce many benefits, including a reduction in inflammation (Toguri et al., 2014). There is no psychoactivity associated with any types of CB_2 interactions.

Although CB_1 and CB_2 are the most well-explored receptors of the ECS, cannabinoids interact with other receptors as well. The transient receptor potential vanilloid type 1 ($TRPV_1$) receptor, which mediates sensations of heat as well as regulates aspects of metabolism, interacts with anandamide (White et al., 2011). In fact, activation of $TRPV_1$ regulates anandamide synthesis (Tóth et al., 2009). Cannabinoids also activate $TRPV_2$. The image on the previous page shows some of the primary receptors activated by specific cannabinoids. As demonstrated, most endocannabinoids activate CB_1 with higher efficacy and CB_2 with lower efficacy (indicated by the >> symbol). 2-AG stands out as equally activating both CB_1 and CB_2 (indicated by the ~ symbol). Anandamide and N-arachidonoyl dopamine are also distinguished by their affinity for $TRPV_1$.

Ligands like endocannabinoids and neurotransmitters can function as agonists, antagonists, or inverse agonists when binding with receptors (Negus, 2006). Agonism means a ligand activates the receptor to produce the standard biological response. Inverse agonism is another form of activation where the receptor produces a response opposite to the standard one, inhibiting the normal activity of a receptor that occurs when nothing is bound to it.

Antagonism is when a ligand binds to a receptor and produces no effect, thus blocking the action of other agonists or inverse agonists.

Efficacy is a measure of how much a ligand activates a receptor. A ligand with high efficacy activates the receptor is a strong fashion, while one with low efficacy does so in a weaker fashion. Interestingly, THC is a partial agonist of the THC receptor, not activating it to maximum effect. This a good thing, as several synthetic cannabinoids which do act as full agonists of the THC receptor can cause severe health problems or death due to their strong activation of CB_1 receptors (van Amsterdam et al., 2015).

Affinity is a different concept from efficacy, and generally refers to the tendency of a drug molecule to bind to a receptor (Salahudeen & Nishtala, 2017). A compound can have high affinity for a receptor, easily binding to it, but not activate it strongly; it would have high affinity but low efficacy. Compounds with low affinity can still bind to receptors, but it takes larger amounts of them than other compounds with higher affinity.

Nuclear receptors are found within cells and include peroxisome proliferator-activated receptors (PPARs). Anandamide and oleoylethanolamide (OEA), the monounsaturated analog of anandamide, mediate neuroprotective effects and lipid breakdown by activating PPAR-alpha (O'Sullivan, 2007). 2-AG and anandamide activate PPAR-gamma to confer anti-inflammatory effects. This receptor's activation also leads to vasorelaxation in isolated arteries. More research is needed to identify the effects of endocannabinoids on other subtypes of PPAR.

There are many other receptors with unknown endogenous ligands. These are called orphan receptors, which are designated with GPR and a number. Several orphan receptors are now being considered as novel cannabinoid receptors, including GPR55, GPR119, and GPR18. Of these, GPR55 has received the most attention, with initial research pointing to energy balance and glucose metabolism functions, among others (Tudurí et al., 2017). Anandamide is the chief endocannabinoid agonist of GPR55; interestingly enough, the plant cannabinoid cannabidiol (CBD) is an antagonist (A. J. Brown, 2007). Evidence suggests that GPR119 works in the pancreas to regulate energy balance. It is activated by OEA and to a lesser extent anandamide (Overton et al., 2008). Palmitoylethanolamide (PEA), another compound with endocannabinoid-like effects, is weakly active at GPR119 (Brown, 2007).

N-arachidonoyl glycine (NAGly), an analog of anandamide, activates GPR18 (Burstein, 2008). The receptor also responds to a synthetic form of CBD known as abnormal cannabidiol (McHugh et al., 2010). One of GPR18's primary functions is directing microglial migration in the central nervous system. Microglia are immune cells in the brain which help protect neurons.

OEA, PEA, and NAGly are not considered true endocannabinoids, but they are endocannabinoid-related compounds that affect the ECS (Caraceni et al., 2010; Burstein, 2008). PEA, several of its analogs, and OEA act as "entourage" compounds to reduce uptake and metabolism of anandamide, thereby increasing its concentration (Jonsson et al., 2001). Several phytocannabinoids also act through similar mechanisms to increase anandamide.

One of the key methods by which endocannabinoids maintain homeostasis is through retrograde feedback. When neurons communicate, neurotransmitters are sent from the presynaptic neuron to the postsynaptic neuron. Endocannabinoids travel in the reverse direction, from the postsynapstic to the presynapstic side, where they bind with CB_1 receptors to reduce neurotransmitter release (Hermanson & Marnett, 2011). This reduction is achieved via inhibition of N-type voltage-dependent calcium (Ca^{2+}) channels. Another mechanism of presynaptic regulation involves activation of G protein-coupled inwardly rectifying potassium (GIRK) channels (Guo & Ikeda, 2004).

Endocannabinoids are synthesized "on demand" from phospholipids in the postsynaptic membrane. They are utilized when neurotransmission needs to be slowed down. In essence, if a postsynaptic cell recognizes that a presynaptic cell is firing too rapidly, endocannabinoids will be released upstream to instruct the sending cell to cease transmission. Recognition is often triggered by increased intracellular calcium levels in the postsynaptic cell. By completing the circuit of cellular communication, the ECS facilitates whole-organism unity. Anandamide, 2-AG, and 2-AGE all exhibit similar levels of regulatory efficacy; each displays approximately 50% maximal inhibition (Guo & Ikeda, 2004). Although these endocannabinoids share efficacy, their potencies are different. 2-AGE is the strongest, followed by 2-AG and anandamide. Therefore, it takes much less 2-AGE to achieve 50% inhibition than anandamide or 2-AG.

Interestingly, whereas 2-AG and 2-AGE rely on the CB_1 receptor to inhibit calcium channels and neurotransmitter release, anandamide can inhibit such channels through a CB_1-independent mechanism (Guo & Ikeda, 2004).

It may be that when an endocannabinoid cannot induce inhibition via one mechanism, another endocannabinoid utilizes a different pathway as an alternative.

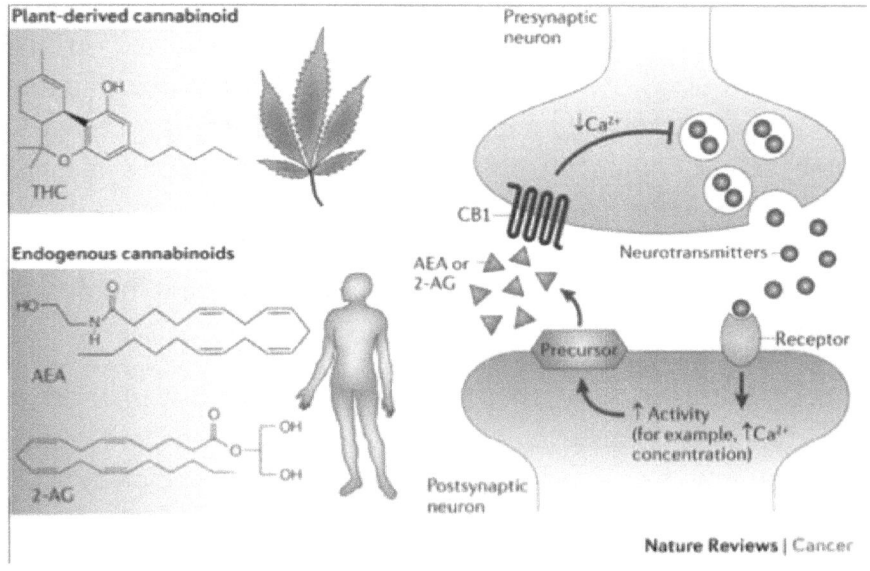

(Velasco et al., 2012)

Research surrounding the ECS is constantly expanding and changing. New receptors and endocannabinoids will likely be discovered as the field advances. The importance of the ECS will also grow, but even now it has already been linked in some way to virtually every disease.

III. THE ENDOCANNABINOID SYSTEM AND DISEASE PATHOLOGY

Scientific studies from researchers around the world have demonstrated the ECS is somehow involved in the pathology of most diseases. Due to this, it is possible that enhancing ECS activity may help alleviate diseases, at least to some extent. When the ECS is functioning optimally, it helps maintain homeostasis, or balance, throughout the entire body. Since all disease is inherently some deviation from homeostasis, it makes sense that targeting the ECS may treat numerous diseases.

Indeed, as the following sections show, there are disturbances in ECS function (mainly relating to cannabinoid receptor and/or endocannabinoid levels) across virtually every major type of disease. Furthermore, numerous clinical trials and massive amounts of media-reported evidence demonstrate that targeting the ECS with cannabis does provide relief for some conditions. It is quite possible that supporting the ECS with other strategies, in addition to or instead of cannabis, could achieve similar results.

Obesity and Diabetes

One of the most recognized functions of the ECS relates to appetite. Most people know that smoking cannabis often increases the desire to consume food, a phenomenon driven by THC activating CB_1 receptors (Koch, 2017). Anandamide and 2-AG also increase appetite through CB_1 receptors, and thus play a significant role in hunger-induced food intake.

Endocannabinoids are involved in both initiation and consummation of eating, interacting with a variety of orexigenic (appetite stimulant) and anorexigenic (appetite suppressant) hormones and neurotransmitters.

CB_1 receptors do more than just encourage appetite; they are also involved in peripheral energy metabolism (O'Sullivan et al., 2021). They are expressed on fat cells, where their activation regulates hormone production and activity, as well as cell differentiation and fat storage. In general, endocannabinoids "regulate energy homeostasis by interacting with central and peripheral targets, including adipose [fat] tissue, muscle, liver, and endocrine pancreas" (Bermúdez-Silva et al., 2009).

Given these properties, it is no surprise the ECS affects obesity. While there are many cases where endocannabinoid deficiency contributes to disease pathology, excessive activity of the ECS (particularly overactive CB_1 signaling) is linked to weight gain (Dörnyei et al., 2023). Endocannabinoids and CB_1 receptors are upregulated in the liver and fat tissues in obese animals. Further supporting the appetite-stimulatory role of CB_1 receptors, giving chemicals that block the CB_1 receptor to mice causes them to reduce caloric intake and lose weight. Also, mice genetically engineered to lack CB_1 receptors resist diet-induced weight gain, even when consuming a high-fat diet.

From an evolutionary viewpoint, the ability of CB_1 receptors to conserve energy is integral to survival. Animals, including humans, constantly faced famine during their evolution. The ability to store energy efficiently, as mediated by the ECS, was necessary. At no point during evolution did organisms have free, almost unlimited access to high-fat and high-sugar foods (Neuschwander-Tetri, 2007).

In this new environment, the ECS's protective mechanisms appear to backfire, storing too much energy and causing obesity.

As this case illustrates, it seems there are ways to "improperly" upregulate the ECS. Given its involvement in so many different areas throughout the body, it makes sense that increased endocannabinoid activity could cause problems in some circumstances. However, directly blocking this activity with drug antagonists has proven problematic, given the widespread function of cannabinoid receptors. A CB_1 antagonist drug called rimonabant was promoted in the mid-2000s for weight loss, but was eventually banned because it could cause severe mood disorders (Sam et al., 2011). Therefore, other ways of modulating excessive ECS are needed.

Curiously, cannabis consumption has been found to negatively correlate with obesity, with cannabis users having lower rates of obesity than non-users (Clark et al., 2018). This phenomenon succinctly demonstrates the complexity of cannabinoid medicine and the ECS. After all, THC-rich cannabis activates the CB_1 receptor, so theoretically it should increase weight gain via appetite stimulation and peripheral energy regulation mechanisms. However, research suggests this is not the case.

Another study using two sets of high-quality survey data found that obesity rates were about a third lower in people smoking cannabis at least three times a week than people who did not use cannabis at all (Le Strat & Le Foll, 2011). This correlation was maintained even after other factors were accounted for, like cigarette smoking, age, and gender.

A later 2013 study determined that current cannabis users had 16% lower fasting insulin levels and a 17% lower homeostasis model assessment of insulin resistance (HOMA-IR) score (Penner et al., 2013). Furthermore, cannabis users exhibited higher levels of high-density lipoprotein (HDL), the good kind of cholesterol, as well as a smaller waist circumference. People who had used cannabis more recently had better measures.

The above evidence suggests that the ECS is involved with glucose regulation and potentially diabetes. Indeed, there are many studies which implicate the ECS in these functions. CB_1 activation has been found to impair plasma glucose clearance, while CB_2 activation facilitates glucose clearance (Di Marzo, 2008). Cannabinoid receptors are found in alpha and beta cells of the pancreas, where they regulate glucagon (increases plasma glucose) and insulin (decreases plasma glucose) release respectively. Unbalanced endocannabinoid concentrations can increase intra-abdominal fat, thus contributing to atherosclerosis and type 2 diabetes. Anandamide and 2-AG are upregulated in non-obese patients with type 2 diabetes.

A 2008 study using CBD further bolstered the ECS's connection to diabetes (Weiss et al., 2008). Mice in a latent diabetes stage or with initial symptoms of diabetes were administered CBD or no treatment. Only 32% of the CBD-treated group was diagnosed with diabetes, whereas the figure was 100% for the untreated group. It is unclear exactly how CBD produced these results, but the phytocannabinoid targets the ECS in numerous ways, including interacting with CB_1 and CB_2 receptors and increasing anandamide levels.

Pain Disorders

Pain is a symptom of many diseases and a condition in itself when it becomes chronic. While acute pain is highly treatable with fast-acting and powerful opioids, there are few options available for those with long-term, chronic pain. The ECS is deeply involved in pain signaling, and its manipulation with phytocannabinoids has been proven to reduce multiple forms of pain.

Anandamide, THC, and CBD can effectively reduce acute pain stemming from mechanical and thermal stimuli, as well as neuropathic and inflammatory pain (Fine & Rosenfeld, 2013). Acetaminophen, the most used painkiller, confers its analgesic effects indirectly through CB_1 activation (Mallet et al., 2008). Endocannabinoids work synergistically with non-steroidal anti-inflammatory drugs to enhance their efficacy, largely via CB_1 activation (Topuz et al., 2020). Not surprisingly, CB_1 receptors are distributed throughout areas of the central and peripheral nervous systems associated with pain (Milligan et al., 2020). Anandamide mainly works through the CB_1 receptor, and levels of the compound increase in relevant brain areas after pain experiences. CB_2 receptors are also involved and play an especially significant role in inflammatory pain (Manzanares et al., 2006). In addition to the cannabinoid receptors, studies have shown the $TRPV_1$ receptor may mediate some of the analgesic effects of anandamide (Starowicz et al., 2012).

Inflammation can be a major contributor to chronic pain. The complex inflammatory immune response to injury can cause tissue swelling, which presses against nerves and subsequently causes pain. Chemicals released during inflammation contribute as well.

Cannabinoid receptors, especially CB_2, are an integral part of immune function. CB_2 receptors are expressed on immune cells; the magnitude of their expression is affected by stimuli that activate the immune system (Cabral & Griffin-Thomas, 2009). The inflammatory response to toxins also increases endocannabinoid levels, which regulate immune function through receptor-dependent and independent mechanisms (Pandey et al., 2009). Specifically, cannabinoids modulate inflammatory cell signaling proteins (cytokines) like tumor necrosis factor-alpha and interleukin-6, as well as many other signaling molecules. They also affect the migration, proliferation, and apoptosis of immune cells. This evidence demonstrates how the ECS is deeply embedded in immune function, and how influencing it could profoundly benefit disorders (including pain) stemming from excessive inflammation.

The ECS works alongside the endogenous opioid system, as interactions between cannabinoid and opioid receptors potentially mediate the effects associated with opioid drugs (Bushlin et al., 2010). Furthermore, a randomized controlled trial which gave exercising participants an opioid antagonist or placebo determined the ECS contributes to exercise-induced reductions in pain responses, and that endorphins may increase endocannabinoids following exercise (Crombie et al., 2018). This and the preceding evidence makes it clear the ECS has an important role in controlling pain.

Rheumatoid Arthritis

Rheumatoid arthritis (RA) is a chronic autoimmune disease that affects joints. Inflammation progressively destroys joints, leading to impaired function and pain. By targeting inflammation and suppressing overactive immune activity, the ECS could dramatically benefit RA.

In many animal studies, various plant and endogenous cannabinoids have been shown to treat RA through anti-inflammatory, analgesic, and immunosuppressive mechanisms. Analgesia is largely mediated through CB_1 receptors whereas immune-related effects are mediated through CB_2 receptors (Milligan et al., 2020; Turcotte et al., 2016). CBD reduces inflammatory markers like tumor necrosis factor-alpha and stops progression of collagen-induced arthritis in mice; THC also alleviates this form of arthritis (Paland et al., 2023). Furthermore, anandamide and THC are effective against general arthritis-related pain. This evidence suggests RA progression may be linked to an endocannabinoid deficiency, and that using CB_1/CB_2 agonists could provide significant benefit. Indeed, a double-blind, placebo-controlled trial found that a mix of THC and CBD produced significant analgesic effects and suppressed disease activity in patients with RA (Blake et al., 2006).

Neurodegenerative Disorders

One of the most important jobs of the ECS is to protect the body from damage, whether it originates from internal or external sources. In general, the ECS contributes to healing and cell protection. Having a strong ECS may even improve survival from head trauma.

Studies show the ECS confers neuroprotection in a wide variety of cases, including acute injuries and chronic neurodegenerative diseases. From traumatic brain injuries to multiple sclerosis to Alzheimer's, the ECS is involved in nearly everything (Calina et al., 2020; Li et al., 2023).

There are a few common mechanisms by which cannabinoids mitigate neurotoxicity, including retrograde feedback (Vaughan & Christie, 2005). In many cases, neurotoxicity is caused by overstimulation of neural receptors by glutamate, an excitatory neurotransmitter. Too much glutamate causes neurons to die; in fact, excitatory glutamate transmission is likely a primary cause of amyotrophic lateral sclerosis, one of the most devastating central nervous system disorders (Foran & Trotti, 2009). Endocannabinoids travel upstream from the postsynaptic to the presynaptic cell, where they bind with CB_1 receptors and instruct the sending cell to stop firing (Vaughan & Christie, 2005). This mechanism can reduce destructive excitatory transmission (excitotoxicity) and protect neurons.

The ECS offers additional protection by influencing neuronal and non-neuronal signaling to an extensive degree. Endocannabinoids modulate the release of inflammatory mediators from many cell types (astrocytes, microglia, macrophages, lymphocytes, neutrophils, and neurons) via CB_1, CB_2, and other receptors (Pacher & Kunos, 2013).

Since excessive inflammation can lead to neurodegeneration, stopping inflammation is a powerful protective mechanism. The ECS activates multiple cytoprotective signaling pathways and modulates calcium homeostasis by affecting calcium, potassium, and sodium channels (Pacher, Bátkai, & Kunos, 2006). In certain situations, the ECS may protect cells by reducing metabolic rate and oxygen demand through a CB_1-dependent mechanism. Finally, a strong contributor to neurotoxicity is oxidative stress, caused by an imbalance of free radicals. Cannabinoids act as antioxidants and can neutralize these radicals. Oxidative stress can result from excitotoxicity, so cannabinoids appear to reduce such stress by stopping it at a source and disabling free radicals directly.

Many of the processes triggered by traumatic brain injury (TBI), such as excitotoxicity, inflammation, and cell death, may effectively be reversed with cannabinoid therapies. Endocannabinoids like 2-AG increase in direct response to injury, as an apparent attempt by the body to protect cells (Shohami et al., 2011). Furthermore, both anandamide and 2-AG protect neurons in the cerebral cortex from glucose and oxygen deprivation as mechanisms of neuroprotection (Sinor et al., 2000).

Research shows the neuroprotective effects of cannabinoids have very real impacts. In one study, scientists analyzed 446 patients treated for TBI, and compared results from those testing positive for THC to those testing negative (Nguyen et al., 2014). After adjusting for factors like injury severity, THC-positive patients were found to have an 80% lower probability of dying than THC-negative patients.

These are incredible results, but more research is needed to determine the effective doses of THC along with the potential utility of other cannabinoids like CBD.

Multiple Sclerosis

Multiple sclerosis (MS) is an autoimmune disease characterized by the inflammation-mediated loss of neural myelin sheaths, which amplify communications. Like most neurodegenerative disorders, MS gets worse as more neurons lose their sheaths and die.

The endocannabinoid system is involved in MS, with one study pointing to spasticity (a common symptom) being controlled by CB_1, but not CB_2, receptors (Pryce & Baker, 2007). two of the most common symptoms of MS. In one study, mice with experimental autoimmune encephalomyelitis (EAE, a lab-model of MS) given compounds that activate cannabinoid receptors experienced reduced neurological deficits and less inflammatory damage (Arévalo-Martín et al., 2003). In another study, researchers observed higher levels of anandamide, 2-AG, and PEA in areas with nerve damage (Baker et al., 2001); like brain injury, this increase in endocannabinoids is an apparent survival mechanism to protect cells.

Further evidence of ECS involvement comes from mice bred without CB_1 receptors. These mice cannot tolerate inflammatory or neurotoxic damage well and have naturally higher levels of pro-apoptotic compounds in their cells (Pryce et al., 2003). In addition, CB_1 knockout mice with EAE experienced greater cell death and more myelin sheath and axonal protein loss than regular mice (Jackson et al., 2005).

These results suggest the CB_1 receptor exerts a general neuroprotective function.

In humans, those with an active form of MS have a higher concentration of anandamide than those with a silent form (Eljaschewitsch et al., 2006). This indicates anandamide may increase as a protective mechanism. The therapeutic effects of cannabinoids are reinforced by double-blind, placebo-controlled trials that have found THC and CBD benefit many aspects of MS, including pain, spasticity, bladder problems, and mobility issues (Rog et al., 2005; Wade et al., 2003). Therefore, it has been conclusively proven that ECS manipulation can improve MS.

Parkinson's Disease

Parkinson's Disease (PD) is another neurodegenerative disorder characterized by impairments in motor function and coordination. It is caused by a loss of dopamine-producing (dopaminergic) neurons, although exactly what leads to their death is unknown. Many of the factors involved in MS, such as excitotoxicity, oxidative stress, and neuroinflammation, are also present in PD (Chakrabarti & Bisaglia, 2023).

PD leads to problems with movement because most of the neurons dying are found in the basal ganglia, an area of the brain which helps control motor function (Groenewegen, 2003). CB_1 receptors and endocannabinoids are highly abundant in these regions. In fact, increased CB_1 binding has been observed in the brains of PD patients, which may be a physiological attempt to normalize function in a dopamine-deficient state (Lastres-Becker et al., 2001).

This theory is supported by the fact that CB_1 agonists confer numerous benefits, including decreasing tremors, reducing motor impairment, and preventing dopaminergic cell death (More & Choi, 2015). However, overactivity of CB_1 signaling may be associated with some symptoms of PD, like bradykinesia (slow movement) (Di Marzo et al., 2000). Different manifestations of PD warrant targeted types of treatments, including appropriate ECS-related therapies.

Amyotrophic Lateral Sclerosis

One of the fastest progressing neurodegenerative diseases is amyotrophic lateral sclerosis (ALS). It results from rapid degeneration of motor neurons in the brain and spinal cord, which ultimately paralyzes most patients and leads to death within 3 to 5 years (Zarei et al., 2015). Studies have shown that cannabinoids can benefit ALS by reducing excitotoxic and oxidative damage, but unlike MS and PD, the neuroprotective effects are apparently mediated by non-CB_1 receptor mechanisms (Bilsland et al., 2006; Raman et al., 2004). The utility of cannabinoid receptor agonists for ALS, including those derived from cannabis, is efficiently summarized in a study by researchers from University of Washington Medical Center (Carter et al., 2010). The authors stated:

"Ideally, a multidrug regimen, including glutamate antagonists, antioxidants, a centrally acting anti-inflammatory agent, microglial cell modulators (including tumor necrosis factor alpha [TNF-alpha] inhibitors), an antiapoptotic agent, 1 or more neurotrophic growth factors, and a mitochondrial function-enhancing agent would be required to comprehensively address the known pathophysiology of ALS. Remarkably, cannabis appears to have activity in all of those areas."

Alzheimer's Disease

The most common form of dementia is Alzheimer's Disease (AD). It begins with the accumulation of beta-amyloid plaque and hyperphosphorylated tau protein, which leads to neuroinflammation and cell death (Rajmohan & Reddy, 2017). There are currently no conventional options for reversing AD, but the ECS offers a promising route of dealing with this traumatic condition.

As with other forms of neurodegeneration, the CB_1 receptor is closely linked to mitigating the underlying biological processes of AD. Anandamide, working through CB_1, inhibits neurotoxicity via numerous mechanisms; it activates cytoprotective pathways and dose-dependently inhibits release of nitric oxide, a molecule which may be responsible for the neurotoxic effects of beta-amyloid plaque (Tadijan et al., 2022; Milton, 2002; Waksman et al., 1999). Interestingly, CB_1 receptors decrease while CB_2 receptors increase in the brains of AD patients, particularly the microglial immune cells (Ramírez et al., 2005; Benito et al., 2003). Endocannabinoids may be released from neurons and glial cells in response to beta amyloid deposition, where they activate neuroprotective pathways via CB_1 and modulate inflammation via CB_2 (Vasincu et al., 2022). These effects were reinforced by a rat study, where administration of a compound that boosted natural endocannabinoid levels by inhibiting their cellular reuptake led to reversal of beta-amyloid-induced hippocampal damage and memory loss (van der Stelt et al., 2006).

The effects of THC, which theoretically could treat dementia through activating CB_1 and CB_2 receptors, were explored in a small study with six patients suffering from late-stage dementia (Walther et al., 2006). Participants were administered 2.5mg/day synthetic THC for two weeks. This treatment regimen proved very effective at improving dementia symptoms, including general neuropsychiatric measures and agitation, aberrant motor, and nighttime behaviors.

In addition to CB_2 receptors, the anandamide-metabolizing enzyme FAAH becomes overexpressed in AD patients (Benito et al., 2003). Too much FAAH decreases anandamide levels and thus limits its neuroprotective capabilities. CBD, which has been shown to inhibit the degradation of anandamide, may potentially treat AD. A study with CBD and AD-mice revealed powerful results (Cheng et al., 2014); Dr. Tim Karl, one of the study's authors, stated, "It basically brings the performance of the animals back to the level of healthy animals. You could say it cured them, but we will have to go back and look at their brains to be sure" (Corderoy, 2015).

Epilepsy

Epilepsy is a term that encompasses a wide range of disorders characterized by seizures. The seizures derive from uncontrolled electrical activity in the brain, but what causes the underlying dysfunction is usually unknown. Given that one of the ECS's prime functions is to inhibit excitatory transmissions, and thus uncontrolled electrical activity, its role in epilepsy is not surprising.

Studies with rats, mice, and humans generally show that CB_1 receptors, anandamide, and 2-AG become upregulated after seizures, suggesting the ECS kicks into action during seizures to try and stop them (Soltesz et al., 2015).

Strong evidence implicates the CB_1 receptor in abolishing and likely preventing seizures. Anandamide has been shown to dose-dependently decrease electroshock-induced seizures in rats via the CB_1 receptor, while blocking CB_1 with an antagonist increases seizure frequency (Wallace et al., 2002). Activation of CB_1 receptors has been suggested to protect against excitotoxicity, largely by inhibition of calcium channels, stimulation of potassium channels, and activation of enzymes.

The use of CBD to treat epilepsy has proven effective beyond all doubt, since the pharmaceutical CBD product Epidiolex was approved to treat seizures associated with rare epileptic conditions like Dravet syndrome and Lennox-Gastaut syndrome (J. W. Chen et al., 2019). In this case, preclinical efficacy of CBD in cell and animal studies translated radically well to humans, arguably even better than the preclinical evidence suggested. Such evidence is mainly focused on simple chemical-induced seizures, whereas CBD has now shown efficacy in far more complex human cases. For several patients, where no pharmaceuticals were effective at all, CBD reduced seizures by 80-100%. While such profound results are not experienced by everyone, the fact that CBD can completely eliminate seizures in at least some patients demonstrates the tremendous impact that targeting the ECS can have. Other plant cannabinoids, including cannabidivarin (CBDV), have shown promise as anticonvulsant agents (T. D. Hill et al., 2013).

Schizophrenia

Schizophrenia has a prevalence of 0.28% throughout the world, and cases have risen significantly since 1990 (Charlson et al., 2018). The condition features positive and negative symptoms, in which abnormal behaviors are present and normal behaviors are absent, respectively. Positive symptoms include delusions and hallucinations, while negative symptoms consist of apathy, loss of interest, and emotional withdrawal.

The involvement of the ECS in schizophrenia is more layered due to the different underlying biological processes behind disparate symptoms. A deficiency in glutamate or dopamine transmission may cause the negative symptoms, whereas overactive dopamine transmission may underlie the positive symptoms (Thaker & Carpenter, 2001; Lewis et al., 2005). Interestingly, overactivity of the ECS could lead to both excessive dopamine and deficient glutamate signaling (Ujike & Morita, 2004; Laviolette & Grace, 2006). The psychoactive cannabinoid THC has been shown, in some cases, to cause psychotic symptoms in healthy individuals and precipitate psychosis in susceptible individuals (P. Miller et al., 2001; D'Souza et al., 2004). There is also increased CB_1 receptor density in certain parts of the brain in schizophrenic patients, as well as higher levels of anandamide in the blood (Giuffrida et al., 2004; Newell et al., 2006).

As with other conditions, it is possible that the upregulation of ECS components is a therapeutic attempt by the body to mitigate neural imbalances. This theory is supported by a 2012 double-blind, randomized clinical trial that compared CBD to the traditional antipsychotic amisulpride.

It found that CBD was generally as effective a treatment as amisulpride, and even suggested the cannabinoid was more effective at alleviating negative symptoms (Leweke et al., 2012). Very few side effects were observed in the CBD group. Patients taking CBD experienced increased serum anandamide levels, which the authors suggested may contribute to antipsychotic effects.

Anxiety

Anxiety is fundamentally connected to overactivity of certain brain regions associated with emotional processing (Martin et al., 2009). There is a high concentration of CB_1 receptors in relevant brain areas associated with anxiety regulation, which suggests the ECS's involvement in controlling anxiety (Tzavara et al., 2003; Pistis et al., 2004). Animal studies have shown that activating the CB_1 receptor can decrease anxiety, while blocking the receptor or deleting it in animal models increases anxiety (Arévalo et al., 2001; Berrendero & Maldonado, 2002; Haller et al., 2002). This makes sense, since CB_1 activation is linked to the calming of neurotransmission. However, in the case of synthetic and phytocannabinoids (mainly THC), there is a clear biphasic effect on anxiety. Low doses generally reduce anxiety, but high doses can actually exacerbate it (Rey et al., 2012; Salviato et al., 2021). This effect may relate to the distribution of receptors in the brain and their varying sensitivities to cannabinoid receptor agonists.

Depression

The initial causes of depression can be varied, but underlying neurological processes factor into virtually all forms of depression. Neurogenesis, the formation of new brain cells, is decreased under depressive and high-stress conditions, so it is possible that decreased neurogenesis contributes to depression (I. B. Kim & Park, 2021).Endocannabinoids and phytocannabinoids promote neurogenesis, and evidence suggests that CB_1 receptors are required for survival of neurons in the hippocampus (Aguado et al., 2005; Bilkei-Gorzo et al., 2005; Luján et al., 2020). Overall, the ECS has been implicated in having an anti-depressant role, and augmentation of the system has anti-depressant effects (Patel & Hillard, 2009).

Some traditional antidepressants appear to mediate their effects at least partially through the ECS. Chronic tricyclic antidepressant treatment increases CB_1 density in the hippocampus and hypothalamus (M. N. Hill et al., 2006). Although it is difficult to determine how much this effect contributes to reducing depression, it appears that the CB_1 receptor does have some antidepressant role.

Increasing anandamide, which enhances activation of CB_1 receptors, produces antidepressant-like effects (Gobbi et al., 2005). Furthermore, the anti-inflammatory effects of the ECS may also be involved in controlling depression (Huang et al., 2016). However, there is the possibility that long-term use of CB_1 agonists like THC-containing cannabis may worsen depression, but evidence is mixed (Feingold & Weinstein, 2021).

Despite the uncertainty, it is likely better for individuals to seek mental health benefits with a combination of THC and CBD, rather than THC alone, as CBD has been shown to mitigate some adverse effects of THC (Hutten et al., 2022).

Hypertension

High blood pressure (hypertension) contributes to numerous health issues and raises the risk of cardiovascular incidents. The ECS may play a key role in limiting hypertension through CB_1 receptors. Anandamide and THC have been shown to lower blood pressure via CB_1 activation (Bátkai et al., 2004; Goyal et al., 2017). Furthermore, the receptors become upregulated in hypertensive rats compared to controls, allowing more targets for anandamide to hit and subsequently reduce blood pressure (Bátkai et al., 2004). As with other conditions, it appears that CB_1 becomes upregulated as a means of countering the deviation from homeostasis.

The impact of cannabinoids on blood pressure is more profound in a hypertensive state compared to a normal one (Lake et al., 1997; Bátkai et al., 2004). In mice and rats with normal blood pressure, both CB_1 agonism and antagonism caused little change (Varga et al., 1995; Lake et al., 1997). However, in hypertensive rats, CB_1 antagonism further increases blood pressure (Bátkai et al., 2004).

Atherosclerosis

Like hypertension, atherosclerosis contributes to numerous other cardiovascular problems, including increased risk of heart attack or stroke. It is characterized by accumulation of immune cells, cholesterol, and fat in arteries, which leads to plaques that inhibit blood flow.

Inflammation and oxidative-nitrosative stress are major components of atherosclerosis. Given the anti-inflammatory and antioxidant functions of cannabinoids, they are promising compounds for treating hardened arteries.

CB_2 receptors are expressed on immune cells in human atherosclerotic plaque (Steffens et al., 2005). In mice, activation of these receptors by THC has been shown to exert a variety of anti-inflammatory effects, including the inhibition of white blood cell movement. The CB_1 receptor does not seem to be largely involved.

Ischemia

When there is restricted blood flow to the heart, brain, or other parts of the body, cells cannot absorb adequate oxygen or nutrients for their survival. Heart attacks and strokes occur in extreme acute cases of ischemia. Previously discussed health issues, including atherosclerosis and hypertension, are high risk factors for ischemia.

The role of the ECS is ischemia is partially illuminated by the effects of CBD, which enhances anandamide signaling and works through the system in other ways. One study administered CBD to mice before induction of coronary ischemia or before reperfusion, which is the restoration of blood flow after it has been cut off (Walsh et al., 2010). Like ischemia, reperfusion damages cells. CBD caused a dose-dependent reduction in tissue death when administered prior to ischemia and reperfusion; it also attenuated the number of irregular heartbeats.

Another animal study examining CBD's effects on a diabetes-related heart problem revealed that it protected the heart by reducing several types of inflammatory and fibrosis-related biochemical markers as well as oxidative and nitrative stress (Rajesh et al., 2010). These mechanisms at least partially underlie CBD's observed ability to normalize general myocardial dysfunction. Furthermore, in human heart cells, CBD protected them from increased free radical damage induced by high glucose exposure. While more research is needed on the ECS and ischemia, the effectiveness of plant cannabinoids demonstrates it must have some role.

Eye Disorders and Glaucoma

One of the earliest modern uses of medicinal cannabis was for eye disorders. Glaucoma is the most well-known of these disorders, and involves abnormally increased intraocular pressure (IOP) that eventually leads to blindness. Significant evidence implicates the ECS in the regulation of IOP. CB_1 receptors and endocannabinoids are found in many parts of the eye, including the retina (Porcella et al., 2000; Stamer et al., 2001). At least one of the purposes of CB_1 expression is to regulate IOP, as its activation lowers the pressure (Cairns et al., 2017). As the referenced study states, "Activation of cannabinoid receptor 1 (CB1), through topical, oral, and inhaled routes of administration of synthetic cannabinoids and phytocannabinoids, decreases IOP in both animal models and humans." CB_2 receptors are apparently less prevalent and their activation has little to no effect on IOP (Laine et al., 2003).

The role of endocannabinoids in IOP regulation was suggested in a study that compared endocannabinoid content in normal and glaucomatous eyes (J. Chen et al., 2005). The glaucoma patients' eyes had significantly decreased levels of 2-AG and PEA, as well as somewhat lower levels of anandamide. The endocannabinoids were found to have decreased in the ciliary body, a specific tissue associated with IOP regulation. Several mechanisms contribute to the pressure-reducing ability of cannabinoids, including vasodilation and retrograde feedback. Furthermore, by acting through presynaptic CB_1 receptors, cannabinoids inhibit norepinephrine release and production of aqueous humors (the clear liquid in the front part of the eye) (Lindner et al., 2023).

The ECS is likely involved in other eye disorders as well. Cannabinoids have proven neuroprotective against retinal neurotoxicity and possess powerful anti-inflammatory effects, making them potential candidates for the treatment of many inflammatory and degenerative eye disorders (Schwitzer et al., 2016). Phytocannabinoids like THC and CBD have been shown to reduce intraocular pressure and preserve the blood-retinal barrier in diabetes, respectively (El-Remessy et al., 2006; S. Miller et al., 2018).

Inflammatory Bowel Disease

Inflammatory bowel disease (IBD) mainly refers to ulcerative colitis and Crohn's disease, which are inflammatory conditions of the intestines. The inflammation associated with these conditions can lead to severe abdominal pain and malnutrition.

The ECS is involved in many functions of the gastrointestinal system, including gastric acid secretion and gastrointestinal motility (the movement of food through the gastrointestinal system via muscle contractions (Pacher et al., 2006). Pain and malabsorption of nutrients are often caused by increased motility, which itself is a symptom of inflammation.

CB_1 receptors are widely distributed across the enteric (gastrointestinal) nervous system, along with anandamide and 2-AG (Cuddihey et al., 2022). CB_2 receptors are also present, including on macrophage white blood cells (which lack CB_1 receptors). CB_1 and CB_2 receptor activation inhibits gastrointestinal motility, although depending on the situation one or both receptors may mediate the effects (Pertwee, 2001; Wright et al., 2008). A clinical trial with a CB_1 antagonist found increased rates of diarrhea in the treatment group (as much as 2.4 times more frequent), suggesting CB_1 receptor blockade increases colonic transit and/or enhances mucosal secretion (Wong et al., 2011). Furthermore, mice with intestinal inflammation had an increased quantity of intestinal CB_1 receptors, which accounted for increased efficacy of cannabinoids in inhibiting motility (Izzo et al., 2001).

Cannabinoid receptors appear to have a general anti-inflammatory role, as mice genetically programmed to lack CB_1 and/or CB_2 receptors experience greater intestinal inflammation than wild-type mice with the receptors present (Engel et al., 2010). In addition, anandamide has been shown to protect against various models of IBDs (D'Argenio et al., 2006). As with other conditions, cannabinoid receptors and endocannabinoids may become upregulated as a protective mechanism.

The effectiveness of phytocannabinoid therapy for Crohn's disease was examined in a 2013 double-blind, placebo-controlled study (Naftali et al., 2013). 5 of 11 subjects in the cannabis group achieved complete remission compared to only 1 in the placebo group. Almost all the cannabis subjects, 10, experienced significant therapeutic benefits, compared to 4 in the placebo group. The cannabis group also reported better appetite and sleep, with no strong side effects. The scientific and clinical evidence has undeniably demonstrated the utility of ECS manipulation for IBD, yet more trials are needed in larger populations.

Liver Disease

Liver disease encompasses more than a hundred specific conditions. The most common sources of damage to the liver include hepatitis C and excessive alcohol consumption, but autoimmune diseases can play a role as well. Liver damage often leads to cirrhosis, which is characterized by the formation of fibrous scar tissue. This tissue inhibits the ability of the liver to add and remove substances from the blood; it also may cause localized hypertension.

CB_1 and CB_2 receptors are found in some types of liver cells (Siegmund et al., 2005). CB_2 receptors become upregulated during cirrhosis, indicating they may play a preventative role in the formation of more scar tissue (Julien et al., 2005). Indeed, mice without CB_2 receptors have worse liver fibrosis than regular mice, and CB_2 stimulation inhibits the activated liver stellate cells which produce scar tissue (Julien et al., 2005; Long et al., 2021).

Endocannabinoids are also present in the human liver at concentrations similar to those in the brain (Tam et al., 2011). Like CB_2 agonists, anandamide confers antifibrogenic effects by inhibiting or killing stellate cells, although the effects are mediated by mechanisms not related to CB_1/CB_2 or $TRPV_1$ (Siegmund et al., 2005). In fact, CB_1 receptor activation may increase fibrogenesis, as indicated by the ability of CB_1 antagonists to inhibit liver fibrosis; furthermore, mice bred without CB_1 receptors experience slower progression of fibrosis (Teixeira-Clerc et al., 2006). Therefore, ECS-related treatments that avoid direct activation of CB_1 are probably best suited for liver disease.

Cancer

There are over 100 different types of cancer, but they all share the similar features of uncontrolled abnormal cell proliferation and potential to spread to other tissues (Soper, 2016; Otto & Sicinski, 2017). In a multicellular organism, individual cells are born with the internal machinery to undergo programmed cell death, also known as apoptosis. When they become damaged or aged, cells will kill themselves for the benefit of the organism. Cancerous cells lose the ability to self-induce apoptosis, continuing to reproduce when they should otherwise die. Strong evidence suggests the ECS is intimately involved in protecting against cancer, and the progression of malignant cancers may be a failure of the ECS to adequately execute its protective role.

The involvement of the ECS in cancer is apparent by the anti-cancer effects of endocannabinoids.

For example, anandamide induces apoptosis in neuroblastoma and lymphoma cells via $TRPV_1$ receptor activation (Maccarrone et al., 2000). The endocannabinoid has also been shown to inhibit proliferation and/or kill prostate, breast, liver, lung, colon, skin (melanoma and non-melanoma), endometrial, osteosarcoma (bone), ovarian, and glioma (brain cancer) cells (Mimeault et al., 2003; Contassot et al., 2004; Hsu et al., 2007; Patsos et al., 2010; Xie et al., 2012; Adinolfi et al., 2013; Ravi et al., 2014; Soliman & Van Dross, 2016; Fonseca et al., 2018; Lin et al., 2023; Akimov et al., 2024). PEA and oleoylethanolamide (OEA), another other endocannabinoid-like compound, also work with anandamide to inhibit neuroblastoma cell proliferation through CB_1/CB_2- and $TRPV_1$-independent mechanisms (Hamtiaux et al., 2011). A metabolically stable analogue of anandamide was found to inhibit adhesion and migration of breast cancer cells via a CB_1 receptor-dependent mechanism in another study, which further stated the ECS regulates cancer cell proliferation in human breast cancer (Grimaldi et al., 2006). Another study found the development of precancerous lesions in mice was associated with an increase in 2-AG, and that increased endocannabinoid levels reduced the development of those lesions (Izzo et al., 2008).

Cannabinoid receptors become upregulated in certain types of breast, liver, pancreatic, and prostate cancers, and likely other cancers as well (Carracedo et al., 2006; Michalski et al., 2008; Caffarel et al., 2010; Ramos & Bianco, 2012; Xie et al., 2012). In relevance to colon cancer, mice bred without CB_2 receptors had more spontaneous precancerous lesions occur than wild mice with those receptors, suggesting these receptors protect against colon cancer development (Iden et al., 2023).

These factors, combined with the pro-apoptotic and anti-proliferative capabilities of endocannabinoids, suggest that the ECS protects against cancer. If healthy cells evolved to develop more cannabinoid receptors when they become cancerous, they would become more susceptible to the anti-cancer effects of endocannabinoids.

The importance of cannabinoid receptors for cancer survival was demonstrated in a 2006 study. Researchers examined the expression levels of CB_1 and CB_2 receptors in liver cancer patients and determined through statistical analysis that patients with high expression levels had significantly better disease-free survival than patients with low expression levels (Xu et al., 2006). In lung cancer patients, those with tumors expressing CB_2 had significantly longer overall survival as well (Vidlarova et al., 2022). This makes sense, as individuals with more cannabinoid receptors have more opportunities for their endocannabinoids to kill cancer cells.

A wide variety of phytocannabinoids, including THC and CBD, also kill or inhibit cancer cells. Susceptible types include: Brain (gliomas), breast, cervix, ovary, colon, lung, gastric, endometrial, liver, pancreatic, prostate, bladder, skin, leukemia, and thyroid cancer cells (Nahler, 2022).

Human evidence also suggests phytocannabinoids protect against cancer. A 2009 study found that moderate cannabis consumers with 10 to 20 years of use had significantly reduced rates of head and neck squamous cell carcinomas (Liang et al., 2009). Cannabis smokers also do not have higher rates of lung or upper airway cancer, despite the presence of carcinogens in cannabis smoke (Tashkin, 2013).

Most importantly, a case study directly linked THC-rich cannabis extract intake to abolishment of leukemic cancer cells in a human patient (Singh & Bali, 2013). Furthermore, a case series with 119 patients tracked over a four-year period found that 92% exhibited some kind of clinical response, including smaller tumor sizes and reductions in circulating tumor cell counts, after CBD treatment (Kenyon et al., 2018).

The ECS is clearly involved in cancer cell regulation, and phytocannabinoids have a definite role in future cancer care. More research is needed to determine how best to treat different cancers with various phytocannabinoid approaches.

IV. ENHANCING YOUR ENDOCANNABINOID SYSTEM

As the previous section demonstrates, the endocannabinoid system (ECS) is involved in practically every major disease. In most cases, a deficiency of endocannabinoids contributes to various disease states, but overactivity of the ECS may be pathological in certain situations. The aim of enhancing your ECS does not always entail upregulating cannabinoid receptors and endocannabinoids throughout your whole body. Healthy practices that support your ECS will improve its overall function, including increasing or decreasing receptors and endocannabinoids where necessary. Ultimately, the purpose of ECS empowerment is to maximize physiological balance, reduce the chances of disease development, and potentially mitigate the symptoms of active diseases.

Most of the following practices relate to non-cannabis methods of ECS enhancement. The use of cannabis as an enhancement tool is discussed after these methods; the plant is indeed a powerful supportive option. However, long-term consumption of THC-rich cannabis appears to be one of the few ways that ECS function could become dysregulated through overstimulation. As described in the previous section, excessive CB_1 activation contributes to pathology in certain cases. It seems very difficult to overstimulate the ECS through non-cannabis techniques. Interestingly, strengthening the ECS through other means may eliminate or reduce the need for THC-rich cannabis for some people.

Nutrition

Nutrition is arguably the most important influence on the ECS's health. Food can either support or challenge ECS function. Avoiding foods that damage the body can greatly aid the ECS by reducing the amount of protective work it must engage in. For example, foods that cause inflammation will ultimately deplete endocannabinoids as they work to reduce inflammation. A diet that incorporates anti-inflammatory meals every day while excluding pro-inflammatory foods has been proven to help with certain conditions.

Diets with a strong anti-inflammatory focus, like the Mediterranean diet, are associated with reduced cardiovascular disease risk (Martinez-Gonzalez & Bes-Rastrollo, 2014). A review of several studies also indicated protective effects against cancer and Alzheimer's (Sofi et al., 2010; Verberne et al., 2010). It is possible that a contributing source of these protective effects is ECS enhancement.

Healthy diets can be modified significantly depending on an individual's preferences. All anti-inflammatory plans include lots of fruits, vegetables, and Omega-3 rich foods like walnuts, flaxseed, fish, and eggs (Giugliano et al., 2006). Whole grains, nuts, and seeds are also prominent, as is extra-virgin olive oil. Meals should be well-spiced with anti-inflammatory herbs/blends like cinnamon, curry (containing turmeric), ginger, garlic, and saffron (Charneca et al., 2023). Refined and processed foods should be avoided, including most Omega-6-rich vegetable oils and white bread, while red meats should be minimized (Masters et al., 2010; DiNicolantonio & O'Keefe, 2018; Papier et al., 2022). Dairy products do not seem to be problematic and are largely linked to decreased inflammation or neutral impacts (Hess et al., 2021).

However, it may be beneficial to replace milk with cultured dairy products like yogurt and cheese, as studies show making this change can reduce risk of Type II diabetes and myocardial infarction (heart attacks) (Furse et al., 2019; Kvist et al., 2020). All the above changes may lead to reduced inflammatory markers and lower blood sugar levels. In general, the following foods tend to be inflammatory:

- Trans fats (from hydrogenated oils) (Oteng & Kersten, 2020)
- Sugar (Satokari, 2020)
- Highly processed grains including white bread (Masters et al., 2010)
- Highly processed vegetable oils (canola, peanut, soy, safflower, corn, etc.) (DiNicolantonio & O'Keefe, 2018)
- Alcohol (Tharmalingam et al., 2024)
- Ultraprocessed meats like salami and hot dogs (Papier et al., 2022)

The effect of wheat, which contains the protein gluten, on inflammation and digestion is controversial. People with celiac disease cannot tolerate gluten at all, but there is also a subsection of the population which is "gluten sensitive" (Catassi, 2015). Anyone actively trying to fight inflammation may want to consider temporarily stopping wheat consumption to see if they experience benefits. There are many high-quality, nutritious gluten-free grains like brown rice, amaranth, quinoa, buckwheat, and millet. There are also forms of wheat which are reportedly less inflammatory and/or more nutritious, such as sprouted varieties like Ezekial bread or ancient cultivars like spelt (Benincasa et al., 2019; Spisni et al., 2019).

While potential negative attributes of wheat are especially debated, the harm of refined grains is generally agreed upon. White grains, including gluten-free options like white rice, are stripped of beneficial nutrients. As noted above, one study found that refined grain consumption was indeed associated with higher inflammatory markers, whereas whole grain consumption did not exhibit this relationship (Masters et al., 2010).

In general, diet clearly affects inflammation markers in the body (Lopez-Garcia et al., 2004). One group of women consumed a traditional Western diet with high intakes of red and processed meat, desserts, fries, and refined grains. The other group with a "prudent" diet consumed high intakes of fruits, vegetables, whole grains, fish, poultry, and legumes. The Western diet was positively correlated with numerous inflammatory markers while the prudent diet was inversely associated with them.

Organic foods may also contribute to a healthy ECS. A variety of pesticides may inhibit FAAH, the enzyme that degrades anandamide, to an excessive extent (Quistad et al., 2001; Carr et al., 2011). Furthermore, research shows organic foods are generally more nutritious than conventionally grown crops, containing up to 69% higher levels of antioxidants as well as lower levels of the toxic metal cadmium (Barański et al., 2014).

Extra-virgin olive oil, mentioned earlier as a significant component of the anti-inflammatory diet, interacts with the ECS. One study showed olive oil and its phenolic extracts could upregulate CB_1 receptors in human colon cancer cells, and this effect may be a novel therapeutic mechanism for treating or preventing colon cancer (Di Francesco et al., 2015).

Evidence strongly suggests that chronic alcohol exposure is not good for the ECS, as such exposure has been shown to downregulate CB_1 receptors in mice (Basavarajappa et al., 1998). A later study found alcohol downregulated CB_1 receptors and impaired receptor signaling, but increased anandamide levels (Vinod et al., 2006). Long-term consumption of alcohol is associated with damage of the central and peripheral nervous systems, which the ECS must work to slow down (Hammoud & Jimenez-Shahed, 2019). Therefore, avoiding excessive alcohol consumption is the safest bet for ensuring optimal endocannabinoid signaling.

Essential Fatty Acids

Essential fatty acids are essential to the functioning of the ECS. Both Omega-6 and Omega-3 essential fatty acids are required for making endocannabinoids (Tang et al., 2023). It is necessary to consume both types of fatty acids because the body cannot synthesize them.

Although humans need to consume adequate amounts of Omega-6 and Omega-3, maintaining the proper balance is critical. Essential fatty acids are metabolized through the same pathways, so eating too much Omega-6 or Omega-3 will inhibit proper metabolism of the other fat (Balić et al., 2020). While overconsuming Omega-3 can be problematic, most people suffer from an excess of Omega-6 (DiNicolantonio & O'Keefe, 2021). This is because Omega-6 is so readily available, primarily in vegetable oils derived from canola, corn, cottonseed, peanut, safflower, and sunflower seeds. These oils are found in a wide variety of packaged and processed foods, so are very abundant.

Most people ingest Omega-3 through eggs and fish, but it is rarely enough to offset the Omega-6 intake. To reverse the increased prevalence of inflammatory and age-related diseases in society, correcting this imbalance is imperative.

Both Omega-6 and Omega-3 fats are important to health, but having too much Omega-6 may inhibit the anti-inflammatory effect of Omega-3 (Innes & Calder, 2018). As of 100 years ago, the Omega-6:Omega-3 ratio was about 4:1, but in modern times it is closer to 20:1 (DiNicolantonio & O'Keefe, 2021). The value of Omega-3 fats are well-characterized, as supplementation has been proven to reduce cardiovascular-related mortality, reduce high triglyceride levels, and improve rheumatoid arthritis symptoms (Kostoglou-Athanassiou et al., 2020; Bornfeldt, 2021; Khan et al., 2021). Furthermore, adding Omega-3-rich fish oil to an anti-inflammatory diet has been shown to significantly enhance effects of the diet on rheumatoid arthritis symptoms (Adam et al., 2003).

Omega-6:Omega-3 ratios exert protective effects across numerous conditions (including cancer, rheumatoid arthritis, and cardiovascular disease) at ratios as high as 5:1, but between 2:1 and 3:1 is more powerful (Simopoulos, 2002). High ratios of 10:1 or greater may promote or exacerbate inflammatory and autoimmune conditions.

Given that Omega-3 fats and endocannabinoids have similar functions, it is very possible that enhanced endocannabinoid production or function is linked to the observed benefits of increased Omega-3 consumption. While endocannabinoids are also produced from Omega-6, an imbalance promotes inflammation.

Most people need to increase Omega-3 rather than Omega-6, but if large quantities of the former are being taken, the latter's consumption may need to increase as well.

The importance of Omega-3 to the ECS was detailed in a seminal study titled "Nutritional Omega-3 Deficiency Abolishes Endocannabinoid-Mediated Neuronal Functions" (Lafourcade et al., 2011). Using mice, the study found that a deficiency in Omega-3 caused presynaptic CB_1 receptors to uncouple from their effector G proteins, essentially disabling them. This dietary-induced impairment of CB_1 function adversely affected emotional behavior. Increased Omega-3 consumption has been linked to upregulation of CB_1 and CB_2 receptors, as well as increased levels of endocannabinoid synthesis enzymes (Hutchins-Wiese et al., 2012). Furthermore, an entire class of endocannabinoids derived from Omega-3s has been shown to exert powerful anticancer, anti-inflammatory, analgesic, and neuroprotective effects (Watson et al., 2019). These effects include increasing the growth of neuronal cells, reducing inflammatory mediators, and killing prostate cancer cells.

Foods like flax, hemp, and chia seeds, along with walnuts, are excellent vegetarian sources of Omega-3. However, the form of Omega-3 in these foods is alpha-linolenic acid (ALA), which must be converted into more potent longer-chain Omega-3 compounds known as eicosapentaenoic acid (EPA) and docosahexaenoic acid (DHA) (Takic et al., 2022). Due to the relatively low efficiency of this conversion, it is important to directly consume EPA and DHA as well. These acids are almost only found in animal sources like fish and eggs. Fish oil is a particularly effective Omega-3 supplement, as long as it is properly manufactured and purified to eliminate heavy metals and other contaminants.

There are also vegetarian algae-based products which provide DHA. Supplementation with algal DHA is likely as effective as fish-based DHA, as it can reduce serum triglycerides and improve cholesterol (Bernstein et al., 2012).

Probiotics

The human body contains an enormous quantity of microorganisms, including bacteria, viruses, archaea, and eukaryotes, that comprise the microbiome (Ogunrinola et al., 2020). Under normal conditions, these organisms perform a wide variety of important biological functions and contribute to general health. Bacteria appear to outnumber the amount of human cells in the body, with one study stating the adult body contains about 30 trillion cells and about 38 trillion bacteria (Sender et al., 2016). The gastrointestinal system is host to many of these positive bacteria (probiotics), where they directly support the immune system. In fact, 70% of the immune system resides in gut-associated lymphoid tissue (Vighi et al., 2008). The ingestion of probiotics from external sources may support digestive, immune, and even mental health. Specifically, studies indicate probiotics could treat diarrhea-related conditions, inflammatory bowel disease, and autism (Culligan et al., 2009; Hsiao et al., 2013). Probiotics also appear to reduce inflammation and may mitigate obesity by reducing lipids and regulating energy metabolism (Kober et al., 2024). Probiotics may even help fight cancer, with one review describing how lactic acid bacteria from fermented foods have been shown to kill cancer cells, reduce proliferation, and inhibit the growth of blood vessel to tumors (Garbacz, 2022).

The anti-inflammatory and immune-supporting properties of probiotics suggest they may enhance the ECS. Indeed, studies do indicate that probiotic consumption can improve endocannabinoid signaling. Interestingly, depending on the situation, probiotics either upregulate or downregulate cannabinoid receptors to optimally benefit the host.

Human intestinal cells incubated with the common probiotic *Lactobacillus acidophilus* demonstrate increased CB_2 receptor expression (Rousseaux et al., 2007). Probiotic administration has been shown to reduce colon pain through a CB_2 receptor-related mechanism, as well as upregulate CB_1 receptors in a species of fish (Palermo et al., 2011). However, in obese mice with elevated levels of CB_1 receptors in the colon, prebiotic administration (which increases intestinal probiotic count by acting as food) decreased CB_1 density and anandamide production, leading to reduced fat mass (Muccioli et al., 2010). This effect is at least partially linked with the ECS' ability to interact with probiotics to augment integrity of the intestinal barrier (Jansma et al., 2021).

Probiotics can be acquired from numerous sources, including fermented foods, drinks, and supplements. Using multiple methods is an effective way to ensure you are consuming high quantities of various beneficial strains. Supplements should contain at least 10 billion colony forming units (CFUs) and be designed to survive digestion. Examples of probiotic-rich foods include yogurt, sauerkraut, tempeh, and kimchi, while kombucha and kefir milk are among the most popular probiotic-rich drinks.

You can also protect your microbiome by avoiding harmful foods. The anti-inflammatory diet described earlier has been shown to improve the microbiome and may help control obesity through this mechanism (Bagheri et al., 2022).

Some aspects of the Western diet, like a high intake of animal-derived saturated fat, are linked to the expansion of pathological bacteria (Devkota et al., 2012).

Herbs, Foods, Fungi, and Supplements With ECS-Related Properties

There are many non-cannabis herbs, foods, fungi, and supplements that affect the ECS. It is fascinating to learn about the diversity of natural resources with the ability to influence the ECS. Several biological terms here, including agonism and affinity, were earlier defined in the first few pages of this book. At the end of this section, recommendations are made regarding what items are most convenient to use in daily life.

- The flavonoids biochanin A (from red clover), genistein (from soybean), and kaempferol (from tea) inhibit FAAH and thus indirectly increase anandamide (Thors et al., 2008; Thors et al., 2010; Zada et al., 2022)

- EGCG, the compound most responsible for tea's health benefits, has a low binding affinity for CB_1 (Korte et al., 2010)

- Curcumin, the active constituent of turmeric, elevates endocannabinoid levels and brain nerve growth factor in certain brain regions, likely through a CB_1-dependent mechanism (Hassanzadeh & Hassanzadeh, 2012). Furthermore, in a rat model of liver fibrosis, curcumin was shown to downregulate CB_1 receptors and upregulate CB_2 receptors, which had a therapeutic effect (Z. Zhang et al., 2013). Whole turmeric herb exhibits binding activity to CB_1 receptors (Yuliana et al., 2011)

- Cocoa powder contains small amounts of anandamide, although it does not appear to be present in high enough concentrations to impart a biological effect (Nehlig, 2013)

- The *Echinacea* genus, including the *angustifolia* and *purpurea* species, contains alkamides/ alkylamides that activate CB_2 receptors with relatively high affinity (Woelkart et al., 2005; Chicca et al., 2009). The compounds also inhibit anandamide uptake and thus increase its levels (Chicca et al., 2009)

- Common black pepper contains the terpenoid β-caryophyllene, which has a strong binding affinity for the CB_2 receptor (Bahi et al., 2014). Furthermore, an extract of black pepper seed (which contains β-caryophyllene) has shown analgesic effects via CB_2 activation (Venkatakrishna et al., 2022)

- Another compound from black pepper, guineensine, has been shown to inhibit the cellular uptake of anandamide and 2-AG, thus increasing their levels (Nicolussi et al., 2014)

- The spices nutmeg and mace exhibit binding activity towards CB_1 receptors (Yuliana et al., 2011). Furthermore, nutmeg extract inhibits both FAAH and MAGL enzymes, leading to increases in anandamide and 2-AG, which may explain the cannabis-like effect high doses of nutmeg can produce (El-Alfy et al., 2009)

- The Vitamin E derivative alpha-tocopherol phosphate modulates synaptic transmission in rodent hippocampus, apparently indirectly through CB_1 (it does not bind to CB_1, but its effects are blocked by CB_1 antagonism) (Crouzin et al., 2011)

- Anthocyanins are found in a wide variety of fruits and vegetables, but especially red and blue fruits like cranberry, blueberry, and red cabbage. The anthocyanins like cyanidin and delphinidin have moderate affinity for CB_1 and CB_2 receptors, whereas peonidin mainly has affinity for CB_2 receptors (Korte et al., 2009)

- Falcarinol is a long-chain carbon compound found in celery, carrots, fennel, parsnip, as well as *Panax ginseng*. It is a CB_1 antagonist and weak partial CB_2 agonist (Leonti et al., 2010)

- Grapes, red wine, peanuts, mulberries, and Japanese knotweed (also known as Itadori tea) contain resveratrol, a potent antioxidant that has been shown to have analgesic effects via CB_1 receptor activation (C. D. C. Oliveira et al., 2019)

- Olive oil may help prevent colon cancer by upregulating CB_1 receptors on the surface of cancer cells (Di Francesco et al., 2015)

- Licorice contains a compound called 18β-glycyrrhetinic acid, which has been shown in animals to produce anti-obesity effects by downregulating CB_1 receptors and inhibiting the actions of anandamide (Park et al., 2014)

- Rutin is a flavonoid found in citrus fruits, asparagus, elderberry, buckwheat, figs, amaranth, and *Ginkgo biloba*. One study found it possessed antidepressant and antifatigue effects in mice via upregulation of CB_1 receptors (Su et al., 2014)

- Flax fiber and flax seed contains a terpenoid compound with structural similarity to CBD that possesses anti-inflammatory properties (Styrczewska et al., 2012; Storozhuk, 2023)

- *Magnolia officinalis* bark is a component of traditional Chinese medicine, and extracts include the compounds magnolol, a partial agonist at CB_1 and CB_2 receptors (more selective for CB_2), and honokiol, a full agonist at CB_1 receptors and antagonist at CB_2 receptors (Rempel et al., 2012). The CB_1 agonist properties of honokiol are at least partially responsible for its anti-anxiety effect (Borgonetti et al., 2021)

- Another *Magnolia* species, *M. grandiflora*, contains 4'-O-methylhonokiol, which can act as an inverse agonist or agonist of CB_2 receptors to cause anti-inflammatory effects (Oh et al., 2009; Schuehly et al., 2011)

- The medicinal herb *Ruta graveolens* contains rutamarin, which has some affinity for CB_2 (Rollinger et al., 2009)

- The kava plant, *Piper methysticum*, contains the kavalactone yangonin, which binds with reasonable affinity to CB_1 receptors (Ligresti et al., 2012). This property may contribute to the relaxing and anti-anxiety effects associated with traditional kava drinks. More specifically, the study proposed that 250–1250mg yangonin may be sufficient to activate CB_1 receptors in humans

- Compounds in the noni fruit (*Morinda citrifolia*) have been shown to inhibit CB_1 receptors and activate CB_2 receptors, with these properties leading to favorable immune system alterations (Palu et al., 2008)

- *Rubus coreanus*, also known as Korean blackberry, was shown to have anti-osteoporosis effects in part due to upregulation of CB_1 and CB_2 receptors (Lim et al., 2015)

- Thujone, a constituent of wormwood (used in absinthe), has weak binding affinity for CB_1 (Meschler & Howlett, 1999)

- The traditional Chinese medicine herb *Corydalis yanhusuo* inhibited trigeminal neuropathic pain in a rat model via CB_1 receptor activation (Huang et al., 2010)

- *Otanthus maritimus*, an aromatic herb from the Mediterranean, contains alkylamides high binding affinity to CB_1 and CB_2 receptors (Rühl et al., 2012; Ruiu et al., 2013)

- A traditional Tibetan medicine called *Melilotus suaveolens*, also known as wild alfalfa, reduced lung inflammation in a rat model by increasing expression of CB_2 receptors (M. W. Liu et al., 2014)

- Sacred lotus, *Nelumbo nucifera*, was found to act as a CB_2 receptor antagonist (Velusami et al., 2013)

- The *Protium* plant species has a terpene called α,β-amyrin with high affinity for CB_1 and CB_2 (Simão da Silva et al., 2011; Sharma et al., 2015)

- The fungus *Eurotium repens* contains auroglaucin, which has good binding affinity for CB_1 and CB_2 receptors (Gao et al., 2011)

- Another fungus, Neocosmospora, contains several compounds (neocosmosin A, neocosmosin B, neocosmosin C, monocillin II, and radicicol) are able to bind with CB_1 and/or CB_2 receptors (Gao et al., 2013)

- A soil fungus, Eupenicillium parvum, contains a compound with binding affinity for CB_1 receptors (León et al., 2013)

- Miconiosides are flavanone compounds from Miconia prasina plants in tropical/subtropical regions of the Americas. The miconiosides B and C acted as weak inhibitors of CB_2 receptors but did not have activity at CB_1 receptors (Tarawneh et al., 2014)

- Betulinic acid, a compound found in the barks of white birch and sycamore trees, among others, is a CB_1 and CB_2 agonist with moderate affinity (X. Liu et al., 2012). Preclinical studies show it has antioxidant, anti-inflammatory, and anticancer activity

- Salvinorin A, a diterpenoid from Salvia divinorum (a psychotropic plant with historical spiritual use in Mexico), has been shown to exert analgesic activity through CB_1 receptor activation (Fichna et al., 2012)

- Celastrol, a triterpenoid from the root of a plant known as "Thunder of God Vine" in Asia (Tripterygium wilfordii and Celastrus regelii), has been shown to exhibit anti-inflammatory and analgesic effects via CB_2 activation (Yang et al., 2014)

- Chelerythrine, from Chelidonium majus (also known as greater celandine), is a CB_1 antagonist (Dhopeshwarkar et al., 2011)

- Pristimerin is a triterpenoid from *Celastrus* and *Maytenus* plants with the ability to inhibit MAGL, the enzyme that breaks down 2-AG, and thus may be able to indirectly raise its levels (King et al., 2009)

- The plant *Zanthoxylum clava-herculis*, also known as pepperwood, contains γ-sanshool, which demonstrates activity as a potent agonist of CB_2 receptors and antagonist of CB_1 receptors (Dossou et al., 2013)

- Sciadonic acid is found in *Sciadopitys verticillate*, the umbrella pine, and is structurally similar to 2-AG. It is able to increase intracellular calcium levels through CB_1 receptor-dependent mechanism (Nakane et al., 2000)

- The root bark of the tropical African tree *Voacanga africana* contains numerous alkaloids including voacamine, 3,6-oxidovoacangine, and 5-hydroxy-3,6-oxidovoacangine, which function as CB_1 antagonists (Kitajima et al., 2011)

- Semiplenamide A, an anandamide-like fatty acid amide from the blue-green algae *Lyngbya semiplena* has a low binding affinity for CB_1 and inhibits anandamide breakdown (Han et al., 2003). Other semiplenamide compounds, B and G, also have weak affinity for CB_1 receptors.

- Another blue-green algae, *Lyngbya majuscula*, contains compounds called serinolamides with structural similarity to anandamide and 2-AG. Serinolamide A has moderate binding affinity for the CB_1 receptor and less-so for the CB_2 receptor (Gutiérrez et al., 2011). Conversely, serinolamide B has higher binding affinity for CB_2 than CB_1, suggesting A and B could be complementary compounds (Montaser et al., 2012). *Lyngbya* algae also contain malyngamide B, which is a moderate agonist of CB_1 and CB_2 receptors.

- Other forms of algae like *Chlorophyta*, *Laminaria angustata*, and *Mycale micraanthoxea* contain endocannabinoid-like compounds (Soderstrom et al., 1997; Sharma et al., 2015)

- Compounds extracted from the sponges *Xestospongia* and *Dasychalina*, including haplosamate A and desulfohaplosamate, showed predominant affinity for CB_1 receptors and CB_2 receptors respectively (Pereira et al., 2009; Chianese et al., 2011)

- Euphol, a triterpene alcohol from the sap of the *Euphorbia tirucalli* plant in Africa and South America, has shown efficacy against neuropathic pain and chronic inflammation through activation of CB_1 and CB_2 receptors (Dutra et al., 2012)

- Some types of shellfish contain anandamide, 2-AG, or related compounds, including mussel *Mytilus galloprovincialis*, the clam *Tapes dicussatus*, the oyster *Crassosterea sp.*, the sea urchin *Paracentrotus lividus*, and the sea squirt *Ciona intestinalis* (Clarke et al., 2021). A number of other invertebrate groups, including *Porifera*,

Cnidarians, Arthropoda, Platyhelminthes, Mollusca, Annelida, Echinodermata, and *Chordata,* contain endocannabinoids, related compounds, or ECS-related enzymes

- The endocannabinoid-like molecule palmitoylethanolamide (PEA) works at least partially through the ECS and has anti-inflammatory, analgesic and neuroprotective properties (Clayton et al., 2023). Researchers have even posited it may be a promising alternative to CBD for those who cannot or do not want to use phytocannabinoids from cannabis

Consuming a variety of the substances on the above list may naturally enhance ECS activity. While many items are obscure and difficult to obtain, a good portion are widely available.

Top Foods and Drinks

- Blue and red fruits and vegetables like blueberries, cranberries, and red cabbage

- Carrots

- Celery

- Grapes

- Peanuts

- Mulberries

- Olives/Olive oil

- Citrus fruits

- Asparagus

- Elderberry

- Buckwheat

- Figs

- Amaranth

- Soybeans

- Flaxseed

- Cocoa/Cacao/Dark chocolate

- Fennel

- Parsnip

- Green tea

- Red wine

Top Spices and Herbs

- Black pepper

- Turmeric

- Nutmeg

- Mace

- *Echinacea* (*angustifolia* or *purpurea*)

- Red clover

- Licorice

- *Panax ginseng*

- *Ginkgo biloba*

Top Supplements

- *Magnolia officinalis* extract or honokiol

- Palmitoylethanolamide

- Vitamin E (alpha-tocopherol phosphate)

- *Ruta graveolens*

- Kava extract

- Noni fruit extract

Reducing Stress and Depression

The mind is intimately connected to the body, and science has proven that one's mindset, attitude, and thoughts affect physiological processes. Therefore, a critical part of being healthy is keeping stress levels low and thinking positively. The ECS plays a major role in the stress response. It maintains hypothalamic-pituitary-adrenal (HPA) axis homeostasis through multiple mechanisms, including glucocorticoid regulation (Riebe & Wotjak, 2011). Endocannabinoid signaling both activates and terminates the HPA axis response to acute and chronic stress (M. N. Hill et al., 2010).

During stress, endocannabinoids are recruited by stress hormones to modulate various cognitive functions. If chronic stress depletes the ECS through over-recruitment of endocannabinoids, that would partially explain the propensity of stress to aggravate or even cause diseases.

High Omega-6:Omega-3 ratios increase the risk for inflammatory diseases as well as depression. Depressive symptoms exacerbate the inflammation caused by these high ratios; as depression increases, inflammatory markers increase as well (Kiecolt-Glaser et al., 2007). Epidemiological and other studies suggest that Omega-3 deficiency may directly cause some types of depression (Kiecolt-Glaser, 2010). On average, depressed patients have lower plasma levels of Omega-3 than non-depressed patients, and Omega-3 supplementation can produce therapeutic benefits. The ability of Omega-3 to reduce inflammation, potentially via ECS-related mechanisms, may effectively treat depression.

While Omega-3 supplementation may be effective for reducing depression and enhancing the ECS, using other techniques to alleviate stress is also important.

- Aromatherapy is an effective stress management method for students (Seo, 2009)

- Certain kinds of music may trigger stress-reducing effects, but the variation between individuals is high (Cervellin & Lippi, 2011). It is important for people to find the music that is most relaxing for them

- Laughter has been shown to reduce stress in postpartum women (Shin et al., 2011). These clinical results support the general notion that laughter is therapeutically beneficial

- A double-blind, placebo-controlled study demonstrated six weeks of black tea consumption reduces the stress hormone cortisol and leads to greater relaxation (Steptoe et al., 2007)

- Touch massage significantly decreases heart rate, cortisol, and insulin levels, indicating a reduced stress response (Lindgren et al., 2010)

- Midday naps after sleep restriction can reduce stress levels and alleviate other problems caused by a lack of sleep (Faraut et al., 2011)

- Art therapy may be an effective add-on treatment to alleviate the stress component of some conditions, including dementia, PTSD, depression, anxiety, cognitive impairment, schizophrenia, and autism (Mimica & Kalinić, 2011; Avrahami, 2005, Hu et al., 2021).

- Activities like walking, reading, and Tai Chi may reduce mental and emotional stress (Jin, 1992).

Yoga and Meditation

The practices of yoga and meditation have been used for thousands of years, and it is only now that science is catching up to the long-reported health benefits.

Breathing is a major component of meditation, and deep breathing alone has been shown to reduce cortisol levels (Cea Ugarte et al., 2010). Chronically high cortisol levels suppress immune system function and cause insulin resistance, which can lead to inflammation (Wilson et al., 2023). Excessive cortisol probably impairs the ECS given the system's close relationship to the immune system.

Meditation-like practices known as mindfulness-based stress reduction and mindfulness-based cognitive therapy, along with Zen meditation itself, have broad-spectrum antidepressant and antianxiety effects (Marchand, 2012). They also contribute to general psychological health and improved stress management.

Incredibly, mindfulness meditation can positively influence gene expression with the effect of reducing inflammation, potentially combating chronic inflammatory disorders (Kaliman et al., 2014). Due in part to anti-inflammatory effects, meditation may benefit diseases like fibromyalgia, diabetes, and hypertension (Jamil et al., 2023). Over time, meditation also induces physical brain changes. For example, meditation reduces the size of the amygdala, which is associated with fear, and increases cortical thickness in brain regions associated with attention and sensory processing (Lazar et al., 2005; Taren et al., 2013). Meditation may even offset age-related cortical thinning. These physical changes enhance stress resilience and may benefit other disorders.

It doesn't take long to see results - according to a systematic review, just 8 weeks of mindfulness-based stress reduction can produce positive functional and structural changes (Gotink et al., 2016).

Yoga breathing, known as pranayama, has been shown to synergistically enhance the effects of meditation (R. P. Brown & Gerbarg, 2009). Clinical evidence suggests yoga breathing may treat depression, anxiety, and post-traumatic stress disorder. Yoga itself is fundamentally a combination of meditation and exercise, employing a variety of stretches that range from relaxing to incredibly challenging. Yogic exercises have been shown to reduce life stress and blood glucose levels (S. D. Kim, 2014). By combining these exercises with traditional meditation, truly immense benefits may be realized.

The scope of meditative and yogic practice is very extensive. Any of the top results from a search engine query of "how to meditate" or "how to do yoga" will yield valid instructions. The most simple meditation involves:

1. Sitting in a comfortable, straight position

2. Closing your eyes and focusing on your natural breathing, noticing the inhales and exhales

3. Gently bringing your mind back to focusing on your breathing when it inevitably wanders to other thoughts

4. The mind will constantly wander – this is okay. Every time you bring your focus back to your breath, it is like a repetition (or "rep") in physical exercise, which ultimately strengthens your brain and may lead to profound physiological changes.

Given the proven ability of meditation to modify the nervous system, it is very likely there are also direct effects on the ECS. While there is no solid research drawing this connection, the overall evidence suggests some relationship. The possibility of an influence was strong enough that researchers from the University of Pauda in Italy conjectured that meditation may improve ECS tone, which is essentially the system's optimal functioning (Brugnatelli et al., 2021).

Acupuncture and Massage

Acupuncture techniques and massage have been used for thousands of years to treat specific conditions and benefit overall health (Field, 1998; Goldstone, 2000). Although benefits have been widely reported, active mechanisms have remained elusive. ECS modulation may partially explain how these techniques work.

Acupuncture is the practice of using needles to facilitate healing. A specific form called electroacupuncture (EA) has been proven to influence the ECS. EA is like regular acupuncture, except electric currents are utilized to stimulate larger areas and gain more control over the process (Hahm, 2009).

EA has been shown to reduce thermal and mechanical pain through a CB_2-receptor-mediated mechanism (L. Chen et al., 2009). Blocking CB_2 receptors significantly reduces the analgesic effects of EA. EA can also upregulate CB_2 receptors in inflamed skin tissue, specifically in keratinocytes (the primary cell type in the epidermis) and inflammatory immune-related cells (J. Zhang et al., 2010). In addition, EA causes increased anandamide levels in the applied area.

While the analgesic effects of EA have been attributed to CB_2 receptors, there is evidence the therapy can also act through CB_1 receptors to exert neuroprotective effects. One study showed that EA pretreatment activated CB_1 receptors and protected against ischemic damage through an anti-apoptotic mechanism (Wang et al., 2011).

A recent review suggested regular acupuncture can activate CB_1 and CB_2 receptors, with the overall effect of alleviating various types of pain (W. H. Liu et al., 2024). This research is supported by an earlier case report, which described a woman with chronic neuropathic pain from multiple sclerosis who used acupuncture and the endocannabinoid-like molecule PEA to improve her condition (Kopsky & Hesselink, 2012). Acupuncture alone was partly and temporarily effective in reducing pain; however, adding PEA significantly enhanced pain relief and lessened the amount of required acupuncture sessions. Both acupuncture and PEA influenced activated glial cells.

Osteopathic manipulative treatment (OMT) involves hands-on manipulation of the body to alleviate symptoms of conditions and increase systemic homeostasis (Roberts et al., 2022). A super-review of systematic reviews found that OMT was most potentially effective for treating musculoskeletal disorders (Bagagiolo et al., 2022). The ability of OMT to modify ECS components may underlie some efficacy, as a double-blind, controlled trial found that OMT increased anandamide levels by 168%, decreased oleoylethanolamide levels by 27%, and did not change 2-AG levels (McPartland et al., 2005).

Other forms of massage may also convey benefits mediated through the ECS.

Massage therapy has been linked to reduced stress levels in cancer patients, and these effects can extend to anyone (Keir, 2011; Taylor et al., 2014). Swedish massage therapy can reduce blood pressure, heart rate, and inflammatory markers in hypertensive women (Supa'at et al., 2013); chair massage improves anxiety in individuals withdrawing from drugs (Black et al., 2010); shiatsu massage reduces pain in burn patients (Ardabili et al., 2014).

Exercise

Overwhelming evidence has conclusively confirmed the immense benefits of exercise/physical activity, including reducing chronic disease and extending life (Anderson & Durstine, 2019). Given the relationship between the ECS and wellness, the influence of exercise on the system is expected. To start, one study reported that exercise activates the ECS (Sparling et al., 2003). Running or cycling for 45 minutes was associated with increased endocannabinoid levels, a phenomenon which partially underlies exercise-induced analgesia and "runner's high" (Matei et al., 2023). Another study showed 60 minutes of intense cycling increase anandamide, but not 2-AG, levels (Heyman et al., 2012).

Exercise has recently been linked to improvements in the brain, which can lead to better cognition and antidepressant effects. A key protein believed to induce these exercise-associated cognitive improvements is brain-derived neurotrophic factor (BDNF), which increases after strenuous exercise (Szuhany et al., 2015).

The previous study posited that anandamide is a middleman in the exercise-BDNF relationship; exercise increase anandamide, which increases BDNF to exert pro-cognitive effects (Heyman et al., 2012).

Overall, physical activity is correlated with higher endocannabinoid levels and increased levels of CB_1 receptors in the brain, which results in antidepressant effects, better memory, more neuroplasticity, and less neuroinflammation (Charytoniuk et al., 2020).

Exercising at a reasonably high intensity is important for maximizing effects on the ECS. In a comparison study between running and walking, those who ran for 45 minutes exhibited higher levels of plasma endocannabinoids, increased euphoria, and decreased anxiety compared to those who walked (Siebers et al., 2021). Interestingly, researchers administered an opioid-receptor blocker to see if the effects depended on opioid-receptor activation, which they did not, further indicating the "runner's high" effect was indeed dependent on endocannabinoids.

Since not everyone likes to run, it is good to see that hiking can also be effective. Both high and low-altitude hiking have been linked to increased anandamide production (Feuerecker et al., 2012).

The importance of exercise cannot be overstated. It sustains and improves quality of life, and is associated with delaying the onset of at least 40 chronic diseases (Ruegsegger & Booth, 2018). Exercise also helps improve psychological well-being at work, thus leading to better performance and potentially overall happiness (Gil-Beltrán et al., 2020).

Cannabis

The cannabis plant produces phytocannabinoids which are similar in structure to the endocannabinoids made by our bodies. Assessing the consistent effects of cannabis on health or the ECS is difficult because of the plant's complexity. Various types of cannabis contain different levels of tetrahydrocannabinol (THC), cannabidiol (CBD), other cannabinoids, terpenoids, flavonoids, and yet more constituents. Many of these compounds interact directly or indirectly with the ECS. For example, THC activates CB_1 and CB_2 receptors, while CBD blocks them (Pertwee, 2008). However, CBD can increase anandamide levels in humans, thus indirectly activating cannabinoid receptors (Leweke et al., 2012). The utility of cannabis to enhance the ECS may include direct substitution of endocannabinoid functions and other indirect supportive functions.

Some isolated cannabinoids have been studied for their effects on the ECS. Short-term use of THC has been linked to upregulation of CB_1 receptors in certain brain regions like the cerebellum and hippocampus (Romero et al., 1995; Zhuang et al., 1998). There is also a bidirectional potentiation relationship between THC and endocannabinoids, with THC being able to enhance analgesic effects of endocannabinoids and vice versa (Suplita et al., 2008). However, chronic THC use has been linked with decreased CB_1 density and impaired cannabinoid signaling (Romero et al., 1995; Breivogel et al., 1999; Suplita et al., 2008).

The rate and magnitude of CB_1 downregulation varies by brain region and in some places is unchanged. Levels of endocannabinoids like anandamide and 2-AG are relatively unaffected by chronic THC use, although anandamide increases can occur in the limbic forebrain (Di Marzo et al., 2000).

Indeed, administration of THC can stimulate the biosynthesis of anandamide by mobilizing its precursor compound arachidonic acid (Burstein & Hunter, 1995). Although chronic cannabis consumption is associated with CB_1 downregulation, this effect can be reversed after four weeks of cannabis abstinence (Hirvonen et al., 2012).

The impact of long-term CBD use is unknown, but likely carries far less risk than high-dose long-term THC use. CBD is non-intoxicating (not causing a "high") and usually does not cause THC-associated impairments, although exceptionally large doses (hundreds to thousands of milligrams) can increase some impairment metrics associated with low-dose THC (Hayakawa et al., 2008).

High-dose CBD combined with low-dose THC can upregulate CB_1 expression in the hippocampus and hypothalamus (Atakan, 2012). Furthermore, one study showed THC impaired learning without affecting neurogenesis (the creation of new brain cells), while CBD did not impair learning and increased neurogenesis through a CB_1-dependent mechanism (Wolf et al., 2010). CBD has also been demonstrated to confer anti-anxiety effects in chronically stressed mice through enhanced neurogenesis (Campos et al., 2013). Some of these benefits may stem from CBD's ability to increase anandamide levels by inhibiting the compound's uptake and breakdown (Bisogno et al., 2001; De Petrocellis et al., 2011). Enhanced anandamide signaling is thought to account for CBD's therapeutic benefits in schizophrenia, so it may explain other healing effects as well (Leweke et al., 2012).

Other cannabinoids can increase anandamide via inhibiting its uptake, including cannabigerol (CBG) and cannabichromene (CBC), which are actually more potent in this respect than CBD (De Petrocellis et al., 2011). A variety of other neutral (decarboxylated, heated) and acid (carboxylated, raw, unheated) cannabinoids, including cannabigevarin (CBGV), tetrahydrocannabidivarin (THCV), tetrahydrocannabinolic acid (THCA), and cannabidiolic acid (CBDA), exert a range of complex effects on the ECS. The complexity is increased given that humans normally consume whole-plant extracts with several cannabinoids present in varying quantities. Thankfully, such extracts have been proven to enhance the ECS and are often more potent than isolated cannabinoids, including for inhibiting anandamide uptake (De Petrocellis et al., 2011). Interestingly, cannabis extracts, but not isolated cannabinoids, have been shown to inhibit MAGL, the enzyme that degrades 2-AG. In this way, whole-plant extracts can effectively augment both anandamide and 2-AG concentrations.

Evidence suggests that long-term, continuous consumption of THC-rich cannabis is not optimal for ECS function and is associated with learning and memory impairments, although causality has not been established (Kroon et al., 2020). Use of low-THC cannabis with significant amounts of non-intoxicating cannabinoids is probably okay, and there appears to be no research indicating harms from long-term consumption of CBD or other non-THC cannabinoids. While this does not mean adverse effects don't exist, the overall evidence suggests harm is unlikely at moderate doses. However, when it comes to treating diseases, employing higher levels of THC is usually warranted, at least temporarily.

There is little research on what cannabis doses are ideal for healthy people, but 10 to 50 milligrams daily of a full-spectrum (containing small amounts of THC and other cannabinoids) CBD-rich product is probably a good level to aim for. Some evidence shows that low levels of THC, such as a few milligrams, can confer neuroprotective and cardioprotective benefits (Waldman et al., 2013; Fishbein-Kaminietsky et al., 2014). Evidence suggests CBD also possesses these properties (N. M. C. Oliveira et al., 2022; Hernández-Suárez et al., 2024).

Any cannabis products used should be lab-tested to confirm cannabinoid content and safety metrics, including absence of pesticides, bacteria/fungi, heavy metals, and residual solvents. This has become mostly standard practice nowadays, but it's still important to check for. The most convenient products are cannabis infused oils, where CBD and other cannabinoids are suspended in medium-chain triglyceride (MCT) or olive oil.

Eating a high-fat meal 30 minutes before cannabis dosing is ideal because it increases absorption (Crockett et al., 2020). Furthermore, the best way to use cannabis infused oils is to let them sit under the tongue for at least 1-2 minutes, rather than swallowing immediately. This is important because sublingual absorption is more efficient than ingestion from foods or capsules, with bioavailability (the amount that gets absorbed in the bloodstream) at 12-35% for sublingual compared to 9-13% with oral (Hossain et al., 2023).

Regardless of what kind of CBD product you have, you can achieve any target dose if you know the concentration of the product. For example, some CBD infused oils are 50 milligrams per milliliter (50mg/mL) – in every 1 milliliter of the oil, there is 50mg of CBD.

Therefore, if you wanted to take 50mg CBD, you would just take 1mL of oil. 100mg would require taking 2mL. The formal way to determine the amount taken is:

Target Dose / Concentration of Product = Amount Taken

Therefore, if you had a target dose of 20mg with the same 50mg/mL oil, the amount taken would be:

20mg / 50mg/mL = 0.4mL

If you had a less concentrated CBD oil that was only 10mg/mL, you would need to take a lot more to achieve that same 20mg target dose.

20mg / 10mg/mL = 2mL

As a final example, let's say you had a target dose of 75mg with a 30mg/mL CBD oil.

75mg / 30mg/mL = 2.5mL

As you can see, this formula empowers you to dose accurately if you have concentration information. Furthermore, most droppers have graduated markers on them that show 0.25mL, 0.5mL, 0.75mL, and 1mL levels.

The number of individual drops per milliliter varies slightly between oils, but a reasonable median is 30 drops. Therefore, by dividing the concentration by 30, you can know how many milligrams are in each individual drop. This is useful for people who do not need high doses. For example, in a 50mg/mL CBD oil, there is = 50mg/mL / 30 drops/mL = 1.67mg/drop. If you wanted a 5mg dose, then the formula still applies with this alternatively-defined concentration.

5mg / 1.67mg/drop = 3 drops

Quick calculations with estimates are okay if precision isn't critical. If the above concentration were estimated at 1.5mg/drop, then it's easy to go - 1.5, 3, 4.5, 6, 7.5, etc. - as you count towards a target dose. The process gets easier and faster with experience, regardless of which dosing strategy you choose.

V. CONCLUSION

The science of the endocannabinoid system is constantly evolving. We are always learning more about how it maintains general health and influences disease. While there is still more to learn, we know enough to justify the use of cannabis medicine and ECS enhancement techniques. In time, humanity will learn new ways to naturally empower the ECS and treat diseases more effectively.

Top 11 Ways to Enhance Your Endocannabinoid System

1. Consume more Omega-3 fatty acids and less Omega-6 fatty acids. Therefore, increase consumption of fish, eggs, hemp seeds, flax seeds, chia seeds, walnuts, and certain forms of algae. Reduce consumption of cheap vegetable oils, and stick to using olive oil, coconut oil, hemp seed oil, avocado oil, or walnut oil

2. Eat primarily a plant-based diet with as much organic content as possible. Avoid inflammatory foods like refined grains, sugar, processed meat, and Omega-6-rich vegetable oils. Avoid artificial ingredients

3. Do at least 15 minutes of meditation a day

4. Do at least 15 minutes of exercise a day

5. Make time to reduce your stress levels by reading, listening to music, or walking

6. Take a high-quality probiotic supplement and/or eat probiotic foods like yogurt, sauerkraut, kimchi, and fermented vegetables

7. Do not excessively consume alcohol and antibiotics

8. Consider using some form of acupuncture, massage, or osteopathic manipulation a couple times per year or more

9. Do not consume excessive amounts of THC-rich cannabis

10. Consume moderate amounts of CBD, CBDA, and/or CBG through infused oils or extracts. Between 10-50 total milligrams per day is a good level

11. While mentioned earlier, it is worth repeating below the most easily accessible foods, drinks, spices, herbs, and supplements which may enhance ECS activity

Top Foods and Drinks

- Blue and red fruits and vegetables like blueberries, cranberries, and red cabbage

- Carrots

- Celery

- Grapes

- Peanuts

- Mulberries

- Olives/Olive oil

- Citrus fruits

- Asparagus

- Elderberry

- Buckwheat

- Figs

- Amaranth

- Soybeans

- Flaxseed

- Cocoa/Cacao/Dark chocolate

- Fennel

- Parsnip

- Green tea

- Red wine

Top Spices and Herbs

- Black pepper

- Turmeric

- Nutmeg

- Mace

- *Echinacea* (*angustifolia* or *purpurea*)

- Red clover

- Licorice

- *Panax ginseng*

- *Ginkgo biloba*

Top Supplements

- *Magnolia officinalis* extract or honokiol

- Palmitoylethanolamide (PEA)

- Vitamin E (alpha-tocopherol phosphate)

- *Ruta graveolens*

- Kava extract

- Noni fruit extract

REFERENCES

Adam, O., Beringer, C., Kless, T., Lemmen, C., Adam, A., Wiseman, M., Adam, P., Klimmek, R., & Forth, W. (2003). Anti-inflammatory effects of a low arachidonic acid diet and fish oil in patients with rheumatoid arthritis. Rheumatology international, 23(1), 27–36. https://doi.org/10.1007/s00296-002-0234-7

Adinolfi, B., Romanini, A., Vanni, A., Martinotti, E., Chicca, A., Fogli, S., & Nieri, P. (2013). Anticancer activity of anandamide in human cutaneous melanoma cells. European journal of pharmacology, 718(1-3), 154–159. https://doi.org/10.1016/j.ejphar.2013.08.039

Aguado, T., Monory, K., Palazuelos, J., Stella, N., Cravatt, B., Lutz, B., Marsicano, G., Kokaia, Z., Guzmán, M., & Galve-Roperh, I. (2005). The endocannabinoid system drives neural progenitor proliferation. FASEB journal : official publication of the Federation of American Societies for Experimental Biology, 19(12), 1704–1706. https://doi.org/10.1096/fj.05-3995fje

Akimov, M. G., Gretskaya, N. M., Gorbacheva, E. I., Khadour, N., Chernavskaya, V. S., Sherstyanykh, G. D., Kovaleko, T. F., Fomina-Ageeva, E. V., & Bezuglov, V. V. (2024). The Interaction of the Endocannabinoid Anandamide and Paracannabinoid Lysophosphatidylinositol during Cell Death Induction in Human Breast Cancer Cells. International journal of molecular sciences, 25(4), 2271. https://doi.org/10.3390/ijms25042271

Anderson, E., & Durstine, J. L. (2019). Physical activity, exercise, and chronic diseases: A brief review. Sports medicine and health science, 1(1), 3–10. https://doi.org/10.1016/j.smhs.2019.08.006

Ardabili, F. M., Purhajari, S., Najafi Ghezeljeh, T., & Haghani, H. (2014). The effect of shiatsu massage on pain reduction in burn patients. World journal of plastic surgery, 3(2), 115–118.

Arévalo, C., de Miguel, R., & Hernández-Tristán, R. (2001). Cannabinoid effects on anxiety-related behaviours and hypothalamic neurotransmitters. Pharmacology, biochemistry, and behavior, 70(1), 123–131. https://doi.org/10.1016/s0091-3057(01)00578-0

Arévalo-Martín, A., Vela, J. M., Molina-Holgado, E., Borrell, J., & Guaza, C. (2003). Therapeutic action of cannabinoids in a murine model of multiple sclerosis. The Journal of neuroscience : the official journal of the Society for Neuroscience, 23(7), 2511–2516. https://doi.org/10.1523/JNEUROSCI.23-07-02511.2003

Atakan Z. (2012). Cannabis, a complex plant: different compounds and different effects on individuals. Therapeutic advances in psychopharmacology, 2(6), 241–254. https://doi.org/10.1177/2045125312457586

Avrahami D. (2005). Visual art therapy's unique contribution in the treatment of post-traumatic stress disorders. Journal of trauma & dissociation : the official journal of the International Society for the Study of Dissociation (ISSD), 6(4), 5–38. https://doi.org/10.1300/j229v06n04_02

Bagagiolo, D., Rosa, D., & Borrelli, F. (2022). Efficacy and safety of osteopathic manipulative treatment: an overview of systematic reviews. BMJ open, 12(4), e053468. https://doi.org/10.1136/bmjopen-2021-053468

Bagheri, S., Zolghadri, S., & Stanek, A. (2022). Beneficial Effects of Anti-Inflammatory Diet in Modulating Gut Microbiota and Controlling Obesity. Nutrients, 14(19),3985. https://doi.org/10.3390/nu14193985

Bahi, A., Al Mansouri, S., Al Memari, E., Al Ameri, M., Nurulain, S. M., & Ojha, S. (2014). β-Caryophyllene, a CB2 receptor agonist produces multiple behavioral changes relevant to anxiety and depression in mice. Physiology & behavior, 135, 119–124. https://doi.org/10.1016/j.physbeh.2014.06.003

Baker, D., Pryce, G., Croxford, J. L., Brown, P., Pertwee, R. G., Makriyannis, A., Khanolkar, A., Layward, L., Fezza, F., Bisogno, T., & Di Marzo, V. (2001). Endocannabinoids control spasticity in a multiple sclerosis model. FASEB journal : official publication of the Federation of American Societies for Experimental Biology, 15(2), 300–302. https://doi.org/10.1096/fj.00-0399fje

Balić, A., Vlašić, D., Žužul, K., Marinović, B., & Bukvić Mokos, Z. (2020). Omega-3 Versus Omega-6 Polyunsaturated Fatty Acids in the Prevention and Treatment of Inflammatory Skin Diseases. International journal of molecular sciences, 21(3), 741. https://doi.org/10.3390/ijms21030741

Barański, M., Srednicka-Tober, D., Volakakis, N., Seal, C., Sanderson, R., Stewart, G. B., Benbrook, C., Biavati, B., Markellou, E., Giotis, C., Gromadzka-Ostrowska, J., Rembiałkowska, E., Skwarło- Sońta, K., Tahvonen, R., Janovská, D., Niggli, U., Nicot, P., & Leifert, C. (2014). Higher antioxidant and lower cadmium concentrations and lower incidence of pesticide residues in organically grown crops: a systematic literature review and meta-analyses. *The British journal of nutrition*, 112(5), 794–811. https://doi.org/10.1017/S0007114514001366

Basavarajappa, B. S., Cooper, T. B., & Hungund, B. L. (1998). Chronic ethanol administration down- regulates cannabinoid receptors in mouse brain synaptic plasma membrane. *Brain research*, 793(1-2), 212–218. https://doi.org/10.1016/s0006-8993(98)00175-9

Bátkai, S., Pacher, P., Osei-Hyiaman, D., Radaeva, S., Liu, J., Harvey-White, J., Offertáler, L., Mackie, K., Rudd, M. A., Bukoski, R. D., & Kunos, G. (2004). Endocannabinoids acting at cannabinoid-1 receptors regulate cardiovascular function in hypertension. *Circulation*, 110(14), 1996–2002. https://doi.org/10.1161/01.CIR.0000143230.23252.D2

Benincasa, P., Falcinelli, B., Lutts, S., Stagnari, F., & Galieni, A. (2019). Sprouted Grains: A Comprehensive Review. *Nutrients*, 11(2), 421. https://doi.org/10.3390/nu11020421

Benito, C., Núñez, E., Tolón, R. M., Carrier, E. J., Rábano, A., Hillard, C. J., & Romero, J. (2003). Cannabinoid CB2 receptors and fatty acid amide hydrolase are selectively overexpressed in neuritic plaque-associated glia in Alzheimer's disease brains. *The Journal of neuroscience : the official journal of the Society for Neuroscience*, 23(35), 11136–11141. https://doi.org/10.1523/JNEUROSCI.23-35-11136.2003

Bermúdez-Silva, F. J., Suárez Pérez, J., Nadal, A., & Rodríguez de Fonseca, F. (2009). The role of the pancreatic endocannabinoid system in glucose metabolism. *Best practice & research. Clinical endocrinology & metabolism*, 23(1), 87–102. https://doi.org/10.1016/j.beem.2008.10.012

Bernstein, A. M., Ding, E. L., Willett, W. C., & Rimm, E. B. (2012). A meta-analysis shows that docosahexaenoic acid from algal oil reduces serum triglycerides and increases HDL-cholesterol and LDL-cholesterol in persons without coronary heart disease. *The Journal of nutrition*, 142(1), 99–104. https://doi.org/10.3945/jn.111.148973

Berrendero, F., & Maldonado, R. (2002). Involvement of the opioid system in the anxiolytic-like effects induced by Delta(9)-tetrahydrocannabinol. *Psychopharmacology*, 163(1), 111–117. https://doi.org/10.1007/s00213-002-1144-9

Bilkei-Gorzo, A., Racz, I., Valverde, O., Otto, M., Michel, K., Sastre, M., & Zimmer, A. (2005). Early age- related cognitive impairment in mice lacking cannabinoid CB1 receptors. *Proceedings of the National Academy of Sciences of the United States of America*, 102(43), 15670–15675. https://doi.org/10.1073/pnas.0504640102

Bilsland, L. G., Dick, J. R., Pryce, G., Petrosino, S., Di Marzo, V., Baker, D., & Greensmith, L. (2006). Increasing cannabinoid levels by pharmacological and genetic manipulation delay disease progression in SOD1 mice. *FASEB journal : official publication of the Federation of American Societies for Experimental Biology*, 20(7), 1003–1005. https://doi.org/10.1096/fj.05-4743fje

Bisogno, T., Hanus, L., De Petrocellis, L., Tchilibon, S., Ponde, D. E., Brandi, I., Moriello, A. S., Davis, J. B., Mechoulam, R., & Di Marzo, V. (2001). Molecular targets for cannabidiol and its synthetic analogues: effect on vanilloid VR1 receptors and on the cellular uptake and enzymatic hydrolysis of anandamide. *British journal of pharmacology*, 134(4), 845–852. https://doi.org/10.1038/sj.bjp.0704327

Black, S., Jacques, K., Webber, A., Spurr, K., Carey, E., Hebb, A., & Gilbert, R. (2010). Chair massage for treating anxiety in patients withdrawing from psychoactive drugs. *Journal of alternative and complementary medicine (New York, N.Y.)*, 16(9), 979–987. https://doi.org/10.1089/acm.2009.0645

Blake, D. R., Robson, P., Ho, M., Jubb, R. W., & McCabe, C. S. (2006). Preliminary assessment of the efficacy, tolerability and safety of a cannabis-based medicine (Sativex) in the treatment of pain caused by rheumatoid arthritis. *Rheumatology (Oxford, England)*, 45(1), 50–52. https://doi.org/10.1093/rheumatology/kei183

Borgonetti, V., Governa, P., Manetti, F., Miraldi, E., Biagi, M., & Galeotti, N. (2021). A honokiol-enriched Magnolia officinalis Rehder & E.H. Wilson. bark extract possesses anxiolytic-like activity with neuroprotective effect through the modulation of CB1 receptor. *The Journal of pharmacy and pharmacology*, 73(9), 1161–1168. https://doi.org/10.1093/jpp/rgab067

Bornfeldt K. E. (2021). Triglyceride lowering by omega-3 fatty acids: a mechanism mediated by N-acyl taurines. *The Journal of clinical investigation*, 131(6), e147558. Breivogel, C. S., Childers, S. R., Deadwyler, S. A., Hampson, R. E., Vogt, L. J., & Sim-Selley, L. J. (1999). Chronic delta9-tetrahydrocannabinol treatment produces a time-dependent loss of cannabinoid receptors and cannabinoid receptor-activated G proteins in rat brain. *Journal of neurochemistry*, 73(6), 2447–2459. https://doi.org/10.1046/j.1471-4159.1999.0732447.x

Brown, A. J. (2007). Novel cannabinoid receptors. *British journal of pharmacology*, 152(5), 567–575. https://doi.org/10.1038/sj.bjp.0707481

Brown, R. P., & Gerbarg, P. L. (2009). Yoga breathing, meditation, and longevity. *Annals of the New York Academy of Sciences*, 1172, 54–62. https://doi.org/10.1111/j.1749-6632.2009.04394.x

Brugnatelli, V., Facco, E., & Zanette, G. (2021). Lifestyle Interventions Improving Cannabinoid Tone During COVID-19 Lockdowns May Enhance Compliance With Preventive Regulations and Decrease Psychophysical Health Complications. *Frontiers in psychiatry*, 12, 565633. https://doi.org/10.3389/fpsyt.2021.565633

Burstein S. (2008). The elmiric acids: biologically active anandamide analogs. *Neuropharmacology*, 55(8), 1259–1264. https://doi.org/10.1016/j.neuropharm.2007.11.011 Burstein, S. H., & Hunter, S. A. (1995). Stimulation of anandamide biosynthesis in N-18TG2 neuroblastoma cells by delta 9-tetrahydrocannabinol (THC). *Biochemical pharmacology*, 49(6), 855–858. https://doi.org/10.1016/0006-2952(94)00538-w

Bushlin, I., Rozenfeld, R., & Devi, L. A. (2010). Cannabinoid-opioid interactions during neuropathic pain and analgesia. *Current opinion in pharmacology*, 10(1), 80–86. https://doi.org/10.1016/j.coph.2009.09.009

Cabral, G. A., & Griffin-Thomas, L. (2009). Emerging role of the cannabinoid receptor CB2 in immune regulation: therapeutic prospects for neuroinflammation. *Expert reviews in molecular medicine*, 11, e3. https://doi.org/10.1017/S1462399409000957

Caffarel, M. M., Andradas, C., Mira, E., Pérez-Gómez, E., Cerutti, C., Moreno-Bueno, G., Flores, J. M., García-Real, I., Palacios, J., Mañes, S., Guzmán, M., & Sánchez, C. (2010). Cannabinoids reduce ErbB2-driven breast cancer progression through Akt inhibition. *Molecular cancer*, 9, 196. https://doi.org/10.1186/1476-4598-9-196

Cairns, E. A., Szczesniak, A. M., Straiker, A. J., Kulkarni, P. M., Pertwee, R. G., Thakur, G. A., Baldridge, W. H., & Kelly, M. E. M. (2017). The In Vivo Effects of the CB$_1$-Positive Allosteric Modulator GAT229 on Intraocular Pressure in Ocular Normotensive and Hypertensive Mice. *Journal of ocular pharmacology and therapeutics : the official journal of the Association for Ocular Pharmacology and Therapeutics*, 33(8), 582–590. https://doi.org/10.1089/jop.2017.0037

Calina, D., Buga, A. M., Mitroi, M., Buha, A., Caruntu, C., Scheau, C., Bouyahya, A., El Omari, N., El Menyiy, N., & Docea, A. O. (2020). The Treatment of Cognitive, Behavioural and Motor Impairments from Brain Injury and Neurodegenerative Diseases through Cannabinoid System Modulation-Evidence from In Vivo Studies. *Journal of clinical medicine*, 9(8), 2395. https://doi.org/10.3390/jcm9082395

Campos, A. C., Ortega, Z., Palazuelos, J., Fogaça, M. V., Aguiar, D. C., Díaz-Alonso, J., Ortega-Gutiérrez, S., Vázquez-Villa, H., Moreira, F. A., Guzmán, M., Galve-Roperh, I., & Guimarães, F. S. (2013). The anxiolytic effect of cannabidiol on chronically stressed mice depends on hippocampal neurogenesis: involvement of the endocannabinoid system. *The international journal of neuropsychopharmacology*, 16(6), 1407–1419. https://doi.org/10.1017/S1461145712001502

Caraceni, P., Viola, A., Piscitelli, F., Giannone, F., Berzigotti, A., Cescon, M., Domenicali, M., Petrosino, S., Giampalma, E., Riili, A., Grazi, G., Golfieri, R., Zoli, M., Bernardi, M., & Di Marzo, V. (2010). Circulating and hepatic endocannabinoids and endocannabinoid-related molecules in patients with cirrhosis. *Liver international : official journal of the International Association for the Study of the Liver*, 30(6), 816–825. https://doi.org/10.1111/j.1478-3231.2009.02137.x

Carracedo, A., Gironella, M., Lorente, M., Garcia, S., Guzmán, M., Velasco, G., & Iovanna, J. L. (2006). C annabinoids induce apoptosis of pancreatic tumor cells via endoplasmic reticulum stress-related genes. *Cancer research*, 66(13), 6748–6755. https://doi.org/10.1158/0008-5472.CAN-06-0169

Carr, R. L., Borazjani, A., & Ross, M. K. (2011). Effect of developmental chlorpyrifos exposure, on endocannabinoid metabolizing enzymes, in the brain of juvenile rats. *Toxicological sciences : an official journal of the Society of Toxicology*, 122(1), 112–120. https://doi.org/10.1093/toxsci/kfr081

Carter, G. T., Abood, M. E., Aggarwal, S. K., & Weiss, M. D. (2010). Cannabis and amyotrophic lateral sclerosis: hypothetical and practical applications, and a call for clinical trials. *The American journal of hospice & palliative care*, 27(5), 347–356. https://doi.org/10.1177/1049909110369531

Catassi C. (2015). Gluten Sensitivity. *Annals of nutrition & metabolism*, 67 Suppl 2, 16–26. https://doi.org/10.1159/000440990

Cea Ugarte, J. I., Gonzalez-Pinto Arrillaga, A., & Cabo Gonzalez, O. M. (2010). Respiración controlada para reducir el estrés. Estudio preliminar de su eficacia sobre el cortisol [Efficacy of the controlled breathing therapy on stress: biological correlates. preliminary study]. *Revista de enfermeria (Barcelona, Spain)*, 33(5), 48–54.

Cervellin, G., & Lippi, G. (2011). From music-beat to heart-beat: a journey in the complex interactions between music, brain and heart. *European journal of internal medicine*, 22(4), 371–374. https://doi.org/10.1016/j.ejim.2011.02.019

Charneca, S., Hernando, A., Costa-Reis, P., & Guerreiro, C. S. (2023). Beyond Seasoning-The Role of Herbs and Spices in Rheumatic Diseases. *Nutrients*, 15(12), 2812. https://doi.org/10.3390/nu15122812

Chakrabarti, S., & Bisaglia, M. (2023). Oxidative Stress and Neuroinflammation in Parkinson's Disease: The Role of Dopamine Oxidation Products. *Antioxidants (Basel, Switzerland)*, 12(4), 955. https://doi.org/10.3390/antiox12040955

Charlson, F. J., Ferrari, A. J., Santomauro, D. F., Diminic, S., Stockings, E., Scott, J. G., McGrath, J. J., & Whiteford, H. A. (2018). Global Epidemiology and Burden of Schizophrenia: Findings From the Global Burden of Disease Study 2016. *Schizophrenia bulletin*, 44(6), 1195–1203. https://doi.org/10.1093/schbul/sby058

Charytoniuk, T., Zywno, H., Konstantynowicz-Nowicka, K., Berk, K., Bzdega, W., & Chabowski, A. (2020). Can Physical Activity Support the Endocannabinoid System in the Preventive and Therapeutic Approach to Neurological Disorders?. *International journal of molecular sciences*, 21(12), 4221. https://doi.org/10.3390/ijms21124221

Chen, J., Matias, I., Dinh, T., Lu, T., Venezia, S., Nieves, A., Woodward, D. F., & Di Marzo, V. (2005). Finding of endocannabinoids in human eye tissues: implications for glaucoma. *Biochemical and biophysical research communications*, 330(4), 1062–1067. https://doi.org/10.1016/j.bbrc.2005.03.095

Chen, J. W., Borgelt, L. M., & Blackmer, A. B. (2019). Cannabidiol: A New Hope for Patients With Dravet or Lennox-Gastaut Syndromes. *The Annals of pharmacotherapy*, 53(6), 603–611. https://doi.org/10.1177/1060028018822124

Chen, L., Zhang, J., Li, F., Qiu, Y., Wang, L., Li, Y. H., Shi, J., Pan, H. L., & Li, M. (2009). Endogenous anandamide and cannabinoid receptor-2 contribute to electroacupuncture analgesia in rats. *The journal of pain*, 10(7), 732–739. https://doi.org/10.1016/j.jpain.2008.12.012

Cheng, D., Low, J. K., Logge, W., Garner, B., & Karl, T. (2014). Chronic cannabidiol treatment improves social and object recognition in double transgenic APPswe/PS1ΩE9 mice. *Psychopharmacology*, 231(15), 3009–3017. https://doi.org/10.1007/s00213-014-3478-5

Chianese, G., Fattorusso, E., Taglialatela-Scafati, O., Bavestrello, G., Calcinai, B., Dien, H. A., Ligresti, A., & Di Marzo, V. (2011). Desulfohaplosamate, a new phosphate-containing steroid from Dasychalina sp., is a selective cannabinoid CB2 receptor ligand. *Steroids*, 76(10-11), 998–1002. https://doi.org/10.1016/j.steroids.2011.03.013

Chiarlone, A., Bellocchio, L., Blázquez, C., Resel, E., Soria-Gómez, E., Cannich, A., Ferrero, J. J., Sagredo, O., Benito, C., Romero, J., Sánchez-Prieto, J., Lutz, B., Fernández-Ruiz, J., Galve-Roperh, I., & Guzmán, M. (2014). A restricted population of CB1 cannabinoid receptors with neuroprotective activity. *Proceedings of the National Academy of Sciences of the United States of America*, 111(22), 8257–8262. https://doi.org/10.1073/pnas.1400988111

Chicca, A., Raduner, S., Pellati, F., Strompen, T., Altmann, K. H., Schoop, R., & Gertsch, J. (2009). Synergistic immunomopharmacological effects of N-alkylamides in Echinacea purpurea herbal extracts. *International immunopharmacology*, 9(7-8), 850–858. https://doi.org/10.1016/j.intimp.2009.03.006

Clarke, T. L., Johnson, R. L., Simone, J. J., & Carlone, R. L. (2021). The Endocannabinoid System and Invertebrate Neurodevelopment and Regeneration. *International journal of molecular sciences*, 22(4), 2103. https://doi.org/10.3390/ijms2204210

Clark, T. M., Jones, J. M., Hall, A. G., Tabner, S. A., & Kmiec, R. L. (2018). Theoretical Explanation for Reduced Body Mass Index and Obesity Rates in Cannabis Users. *Cannabis and cannabinoid research*, 3(1), 259–271. https://doi.org/10.1089/can.2018.0045

Clayton, P., Subah, S., Venkatesh, R., Hill, M., & Bogoda, N. (2023). Palmitoylethanolamide: A Potential Alternative to Cannabidiol. *Journal of dietary supplements*, 20(3), 505–530.https://doi.org/10.1080/19390211.2021.2005733

Contassot, E., Wilmotte, R., Tenan, M., Belkouch, M. C., Schnüriger, V., de Tribolet, N., Burkhardt, K., & Dietrich, P. Y. (2004). Arachidonylethanolamide induces apoptosis of human glioma cells through vanilloid receptor-1. *Journal of neuropathology and experimental neurology*, 63(9), 956–963. https://doi.org/10.1093/jnen/63.9.956

Corderoy, A. (2015, January 7). *Cannabis May Help Reverse Dementia: Study*. Sydney Morning Herald. https://www.smh.com.au/healthcare/cannabis-may-help-reverse-dementia-study-20130206- 2dxsk.html

Crockett, J., Critchley, D., Tayo, B., Berwaerts, J., & Morrison, G. (2020). A phase 1, randomized, pharmacokinetic trial of the effect of different meal compositions, whole milk, and alcohol on cannabidiol exposure and safety in healthy subjects. *Epilepsia, 61*(2), 267–277.https://doi.org/10.1111/epi.16419

Crombie, K. M., Brellenthin, A. G., Hillard, C. J., & Koltyn, K. F. (2018). Endocannabinoid and Opioid System Interactions in Exercise-Induced Hypoalgesia. *Pain medicine (Malden, Mass.), 19*(1), 118–123. https://doi.org/10.1093/pm/pnx058

Crouzin, N., de Jesus Ferreira, M. C., Cohen-Solal, C., M'Kadmi, C., Bernad, N., Martinez, J., Barbanel, G., Vignes, M., & Guiramand, J. (2011). α-tocopherol and α-tocopheryl phosphate interact with the cannabinoid system in the rodent hippocampus. *Free radical biology & medicine, 51*(9), 1643–1655. https://doi.org/10.1016/j.freeradbiomed.2011.07.012

Cuddihey, H., MacNaughton, W. K., & Sharkey, K. A. (2022). Role of the Endocannabinoid System in the Regulation of Intestinal Homeostasis. *Cellular and molecular gastroenterology and hepatology, 14*(4), 947–963. https://doi.org/10.1016/j.jcmgh.2022.05.015

Culligan, E. P., Hill, C., & Sleator, R. D. (2009). Probiotics and gastrointestinal disease: successes, problems and future prospects. *Gut pathogens, 1*(1), 19. https://doi.org/10.1186/1757-4749-1-19

D'Argenio, G., Valenti, M., Scaglione, G., Cosenza, V., Sorrentini, I., & Di Marzo, V. (2006). Up-regulation of anandamide levels as an endogenous mechanism and a pharmacological strategy to limit colon inflammation. *FASEB journal : official publication of the Federation of American Societies for Experimental Biology, 20*(3), 568–570. https://doi.org/10.1096/fj.05-4943fje

De Petrocellis, L., Ligresti, A., Moriello, A. S., Allarà, M., Bisogno, T., Petrosino, S., Stott, C. G., & Di Marzo, V. (2011). Effects of cannabinoids and cannabinoid-enriched Cannabis extracts on TRP channels and endocannabinoid metabolic enzymes. *British journal of pharmacology, 163*(7), 1479–1494. https://doi.org/10.1111/j.1476-5381.2010.01166.x

Devkota, S., Wang, Y., Musch, M. W., Leone, V., Fehlner-Peach, H., Nadimpalli, A., Antonopoulos, D. A., Jabri, B., & Chang, E. B. (2012). Dietary-fat-induced taurocholic acid promotes pathobiont expansion and colitis in Il10-/- mice. *Nature, 487*(7405), 104–108. https://doi.org/10.1038/nature11225

Dhopeshwarkar, A. S., Jain, S., Liao, C., Ghose, S. K., Bisset, K. M., & Nicholson, R. A. (2011). The actions of benzophenanthridine alkaloids, piperonyl butoxide and (S)-methoprene at the G-protein coupled cannabinoid CB_1 receptor in vitro. *European journal of pharmacology, 654*(1), 26–32. https://doi.org/10.1016/j.ejphar.2010.11.033

Di Francesco, A., Falconi, A., Di Germanio, C., Micioni Di Bonaventura, M. V., Costa, A., Caramuta, S., Del Carlo, M., Compagnone, D., Dainese, E., Cifani, C., Maccarrone, M., & D'Addario, C. (2015). Extravirgin olive oil up-regulates CB_1 tumor suppressor gene in human colon cancer cells and in rat colon via epigenetic mechanisms. *The Journal of nutritional biochemistry, 26*(3), 250–258. https://doi.org/10.1016/j.jnutbio.2014.10.013

Di Marzo V. (2008). The endocannabinoid system in obesity and type 2 diabetes. *Diabetologia, 51*(8), 1356–1367. https://doi.org/10.1007/s00125-008-1048-2

Di Marzo, V., Berrendero, F., Bisogno, T., González, S., Cavaliere, P., Romero, J., Cebeira, M., Ramos, J. A., & Fernández-Ruiz, J. J. (2000). Enhancement of anandamide formation in the limbic forebrain and reduction of endocannabinoid contents in the striatum of delta9-tetrahydrocannabinol- tolerant rats. *Journal of neurochemistry, 74*(4), 1627–1635. https://doi.org/10.1046/j.1471-4159.2000.0741627.x

Di Marzo, V., Hill, M. P., Bisogno, T., Crossman, A. R., & Brotchie, J. M. (2000). Enhanced levels of endogenous cannabinoids in the globus pallidus are associated with a reduction in movement in an animal model of Parkinson's disease. *FASEB journal : official publication of the Federation of American Societies for Experimental Biology, 14*(10), 1432–1438. https://doi.org/10.1096/fj.14.10.1432

DiNicolantonio, J. J., & O'Keefe, J. H. (2018). Omega-6 vegetable oils as a driver of coronary heart disease: the oxidized linoleic acid hypothesis. *Open heart, 5*(2), e000898. https://doi.org/10.1136/openhrt-2018-000898

DiNicolantonio, J. J., & O'Keefe, J. (2021). The Importance of Maintaining a Low Omega-6/Omega-3 Ratio for Reducing the Risk of Autoimmune Diseases, Asthma, and Allergies. *Missouri medicine, 118*(5), 453–459.

Dörnyei, G., Vass, Z., Juhász, C. B., Nádasy, G. L., Hunyady, L., & Szekeres, M. (2023). Role of the Endocannabinoid System in Metabolic Control Processes and in the Pathogenesis of Metabolic Syndrome: An Update. *Biomedicines, 11*(2), 306. https://doi.org/10.3390/biomedicines11020306

Dossou, K. S., Devkota, K. P., Morton, C., Egan, J. M., Lu, G., Beutler, J. A., & Moaddel, R. (2013). Identification of CB1/CB2 ligands from Zanthoxylum bungeanum. *Journal of natural products, 76*(11), 2060–2064. https://doi.org/10.1021/np400478c

D'Souza, D. C., Perry, E., MacDougall, L., Ammerman, Y., Cooper, T., Wu, Y. T., Braley, G., Gueorguieva, R., & Krystal, J. H. (2004). The psychotomimetic effects of intravenous delta-9-tetrahydrocannabinol in healthy individuals: implications for psychosis. *Neuropsychopharmacology : official publication of the American College of Neuropsychopharmacology, 29*(8), 1558–1572. https://doi.org/10.1038/sj.npp.1300496

Dutra, R. C., Simão da Silva, K. A., Bento, A. F., Marcon, R., Paszcuk, A. F., Meotti, F. C., Pianowski, L. F., & Calixto, J. B. (2012). Euphol, a tetracyclic triterpene produces antinociceptive effects in inflammatory and neuropathic pain: the involvement of cannabinoid system. *Neuropharmacology, 63*(4), 593–605. https://doi.org/10.1016/j.neuropharm.2012.05.008

Eglen, R. M., Bosse, R., & Reisine, T. (2007). Emerging concepts of guanine nucleotide-binding protein- coupled receptor (GPCR) function and implications for high throughput screening. *Assay and drug development technologies, 5*(3), 425–451. https://doi.org/10.1089/adt.2007.062

El-Alfy, A. T., Wilson, L., ElSohly, M. A., & Abourashed, E. A. (2009). Towards a better understanding of the psychopharmacology of nutmeg: Activities in the mouse tetrad assay. *Journal of ethnopharmacology, 126*(2), 280–286. https://doi.org/10.1016/j.jep.2009.08.026

Eljaschewitsch, E., Witting, A., Mawrin, C., Lee, T., Schmidt, P. M., Wolf, S., Hoertnagl, H., Raine, C. S., Schneider-Stock, R., Nitsch, R., & Ullrich, O. (2006). The endocannabinoid anandamide protects neurons during CNS inflammation by induction of MKP-1 in microglial cells. *Neuron, 49*(1), 67– 79. https://doi.org/10.1016/j.neuron.2005.11.027

El-Remessy, A. B., Al-Shabrawey, M., Khalifa, Y., Tsai, N. T., Caldwell, R. B., & Liou, G. I. (2006). Neuroprotective and blood-retinal barrier-preserving effects of cannabidiol in experimental diabetes. *The American journal of pathology, 168*(1), 235–244. https://doi.org/10.2353/ajpath.2006.050500

Engel, M. A., Kellermann, C. A., Burnat, G., Hahn, E. G., Rau, T., & Konturek, P. C. (2010). Mice lacking cannabinoid CB1-, CB2-receptors or both receptors show increased susceptibility to trinitrobenzene sulfonic acid (TNBS)-induced colitis. *Journal of physiology and pharmacology : an official journal of the Polish Physiological Society, 61*(1), 89–97.

Faraut, B., Boudjeltia, K. Z., Dyzma, M., Rousseau, A., David, E., Stenuit, P., Franck, T., Van Antwerpen, P., Vanhaeverbeek, M., & Kerkhofs, M. (2011). Benefits of napping and an extended duration of recovery sleep on alertness and immune cells after acute sleep restriction. *Brain, behavior, and immunity, 25*(1), 16–24. https://doi.org/10.1016/j.bbi.2010.08.001

Feingold, D., & Weinstein, A. (2021). Cannabis and Depression. *Advances in experimental medicine and biology, 1264*, 67–80. https://doi.org/10.1007/978-3-030-57369-0_5

Feuerecker, M., Hauer, D., Toth, R., Demetz, F., Hölzl, J., Thiel, M., Kaufmann, I., Schelling, G., & Choukèr, A. (2012). Effects of exercise stress on the endocannabinoid system in humans under field conditions. *European journal of applied physiology, 112*(7), 2777–2781. https://doi.org/10.1007/s00421-011-2237-0

Fichna, J., Dicay, M., Lewellyn, K., Janecka, A., Zjawiony, J. K., MacNaughton, W. K., & Storr, M. A. (2012). Salvinorin A has antiinflammatory and antinociceptive effects in experimental models of colitis in mice mediated by KOR and CB1 receptors. *Inflammatory bowel diseases, 18*(6), 1137–1145. https://doi.org/10.1002/ibd.21873

Field T. M. (1998). Massage therapy effects. *The American psychologist, 53*(12), 1270–1281. https://doi.org/10.1037//0003-066x.53.12.1270

Fine, P. G., & Rosenfeld, M. J. (2013). The endocannabinoid system, cannabinoids, and pain. *Rambam Maimonides medical journal, 4*(4), e0022. https://doi.org/10.5041/RMMJ.10129

Fishbein-Kaminietsky, M., Gafni, M., & Sarne, Y. (2014). Ultralow doses of cannabinoid drugs protect the mouse brain from inflammation-induced cognitive damage. *Journal of neuroscience research*, 92(12), 1669–1677. https://doi.org/10.1002/jnr.23452

Fonseca, B. M., Correia-da-Silva, G., & Teixeira, N. A. (2018). Cannabinoid-induced cell death in endometrial cancer cells: involvement of TRPV1 receptors in apoptosis. *Journal of physiology and biochemistry*, 74(2), 261–272. https://doi.org/10.1007/s13105-018-0611-7

Foran, E., & Trotti, D. (2009). Glutamate transporters and the excitotoxic path to motor neuron degeneration in amyotrophic lateral sclerosis. *Antioxidants & redox signaling*, 11(7), 1587–1602. https://doi.org/10.1089/ars.2009.2444

Furse, S., Torres, A. G., & Koulman, A. (2019). Fermentation of Milk into Yoghurt and Cheese Leads to Contrasting Lipid and Glyceride Profiles. *Nutrients*, 11(9), 2178. https://doi.org/10.3390/nu11092178

Gao, J., León, F., Radwan, M. M., Dale, O. R., Husni, A. S., Manly, S. P., Lupien, S., Wang, X., Hill, R. A., Dugan, F. M., Cutler, H. G., & Cutler, S. J. (2011). Benzyl derivatives with in vitro binding affinity for human opioid and cannabinoid receptors from the fungus Eurotium repens. *Journal of natural products*, 74(7), 1636–1639. https://doi.org/10.1021/np200147c

Gao, J., Radwan, M. M., León, F., Dale, O. R., Husni, A. S., Wu, Y., Lupien, S., Wang, X., Manly, S. P., Hill, R. A., Dugan, F. M., Cutler, H. G., & Cutler, S. J. (2013). Neocosmospora sp.-derived resorcylic acid lactones with in vitro binding affinity for human opioid and cannabinoid receptors. *Journal of natural products*, 76(5), 824–828. https://doi.org/10.1021/np300653d

Garbacz K. (2022). Anticancer activity of lactic acid bacteria. *Seminars in cancer biology*, 86(Pt 3), 356–366. https://doi.org/10.1016/j.semcancer.2021.12.013

Gil-Beltrán, E., Meneghel, I., Llorens, S., & Salanova, M. (2020). Get Vigorous with Physical Exercise and Improve Your Well-Being at Work!. *International journal of environmental research and public health*, 17(17), 6384. https://doi.org/10.3390/ijerph17176384

Giuffrida, A., Leweke, F. M., Gerth, C. W., Schreiber, D., Koethe, D., Faulhaber, J., Klosterkötter, J., & Piomelli, D. (2004). Cerebrospinal anandamide levels are elevated in acute schizophrenia and are inversely correlated with psychotic symptoms. *Neuropsychopharmacology : official publication of the American College of Neuropsychopharmacology*, 29(11), 2108–2114. https://doi.org/10.1038/sj.npp.1300558

Giugliano, D., Ceriello, A., & Esposito, K. (2006). The effects of diet on inflammation: emphasis on the metabolic syndrome. *Journal of the American College of Cardiology*, 48(4), 677–685. https://doi.org/10.1016/j.jacc.2006.03.052

Gobbi, G., Bambico, F. R., Mangieri, R., Bortolato, M., Campolongo, P., Solinas, M., Cassano, T., Morgese, M. G., Debonnel, G., Duranti, A., Tontini, A., Tarzia, G., Mor, M., Trezza, V., Goldberg, S. R., Cuomo, V., & Piomelli, D. (2005). Antidepressant-like activity and modulation of brain monoaminergic transmission by blockade of anandamide hydrolysis. *Proceedings of the National Academy of Sciences of the United States of America*, 102(51), 18620–18625. https://doi.org/10.1073/pnas.0509591102

Goldstone L. A. (2000). Massage as an orthodox medical treatment past and future. *Complementary therapies in nursing & midwifery*, 6(4), 169–175. https://doi.org/10.1054/ctnm.2000.0493

Gotink, R. A., Meijboom, R., Vernooij, M. W., Smits, M., & Hunink, M. G. (2016). 8-week Mindfulness Based Stress Reduction induces brain changes similar to traditional long-term meditation practice - A systematic review. *Brain and cognition*, 108, 32–41. https://doi.org/10.1016/j.bandc.2016.07.001

Goyal, H., Awad, H. H., & Ghali, J. K. (2017). Role of cannabis in cardiovascular disorders. *Journal of thoracic disease*, 9(7), 2079–2092. https://doi.org/10.21037/jtd.2017.06.104

Groenewegen H. J. (2003). The basal ganglia and motor control. *Neural plasticity*, 10(1-2), 107–120. https://doi.org/10.1155/NP.2003.107

Guo, J., & Ikeda, S. R. (2004). Endocannabinoids modulate N-type calcium channels and G-protein- coupled inwardly rectifying potassium channels via CB1 cannabinoid receptors heterologously expressed in mammalian neurons. *Molecular pharmacology*, 65(3), 665–674. https://doi.org/10.1124/mol.65.3.665

Grimaldi, C., Pisanti, S., Laezza, C., Malfitano, A. M., Santoro, A., Vitale, M., Caruso, M. G., Notarnicola, M., Iacuzzo, I., Portella, G., Di Marzo, V., & Bifulco, M. (2006). Anandamide inhibits adhesion and migration of breast cancer cells. *Experimental cell research, 312*(4), 363–373. https://doi.org/10.1016/j.yexcr.2005.10.024

Gutiérrez, M., Pereira, A. R., Debonsi, H. M., Ligresti, A., Di Marzo, V., & Gerwick, W. H. (2011). Cannabinomimetic lipid from a marine cyanobacterium. *Journal of natural products, 74*(10), 2313–2317. https://doi.org/10.1021/np200610t

Hahm T. S. (2009). Electroacupuncture. *Korean journal of anesthesiology, 57*(1), 3–7. https://doi.org/10.4097/kjae.2009.57.1.3

Haller, J., Bakos, N., Szirmay, M., Ledent, C., & Freund, T. F. (2002). The effects of genetic and pharmacological blockade of the CB1 cannabinoid receptor on anxiety. *The European journal of neuroscience, 16*(7), 1395–1398. https://doi.org/10.1046/j.1460-9568.2002.02192.x

Hammoud, N., & Jimenez-Shahed, J. (2019). Chronic Neurologic Effects of Alcohol. *Clinics in liver disease, 23*(1), 141–155. https://doi.org/10.1016/j.cld.2018.09.010

Hamtiaux, L., Hansoulle, L., Dauguet, N., Muccioli, G. G., Gallez, B., & Lambert, D. M. (2011). Increasing antiproliferative properties of endocannabinoids in N1E-115 neuroblastoma cells through inhibition of their metabolism. *PloS one, 6*(10), e26823. https://doi.org/10.1371/journal.pone.0026823

Han, B., McPhail, K. L., Ligresti, A., Di Marzo, V., & Gerwick, W. H. (2003). Semiplenamides A-G, fatty acid amides from a Papua New Guinea collection of the marine cyanobacterium Lyngbya semiplena. *Journal of natural products, 66*(10), 1364–1368. https://doi.org/10.1021/np030242n

Hassanzadeh, P., & Hassanzadeh, A. (2012). The CB$_1$ receptor-mediated endocannabinoid signaling and NGF: the novel targets of curcumin. *Neurochemical research, 37*(5), 1112–1120. https://doi.org/10.1007/s11064-012-0716-2

Hayakawa, K., Mishima, K., Hazekawa, M., Sano, K., Irie, K., Orito, K., Egawa, T., Kitamura, Y., Uchida, N., Nishimura, R., Egashira, N., Iwasaki, K., & Fujiwara, M. (2008). Cannabidiol potentiates pharmacological effects of Delta(9)-tetrahydrocannabinol via CB(1) receptor-dependent mechanism. *Brain research, 1188*, 157–164. https://doi.org/10.1016/j.brainres.2007.09.090

Hermanson, D. J., & Marnett, L. J. (2011). Cannabinoids, endocannabinoids, and cancer. *Cancer metastasis reviews, 30*(3-4), 599–612. https://doi.org/10.1007/s10555-011-9318-8

Hernández-Suárez, Á., Marin-Castañeda, L. A., Rubio, C., & Romo-Parra, H. (2024). Effect of cannabidiol as a neuroprotective agent on neurodevelopmental impairment in rats with neonatal hypoxia. *Brain & development, 46*(9), 294–301. https://doi.org/10.1016/j.braindev.2024.07.002

Hess, J. M., Stephensen, C. B., Kratz, M., & Bolling, B. W. (2021). Exploring the Links between Diet and Inflammation: Dairy Foods as Case Studies. *Advances in nutrition (Bethesda, Md.), 12*(Suppl 1), 1S–13S. https://doi.org/10.1093/advances/nmab108

Heyman, E., Gamelin, F. X., Goekint, M., Piscitelli, F., Roelands, B., Leclair, E., Di Marzo, V., & Meeusen, R. (2012). Intense exercise increases circulating endocannabinoid and BDNF levels in humans-- possible implications for reward and depression. *Psychoneuroendocrinology, 37*(6), 844–851. https://doi.org/10.1016/j.psyneuen.2011.09.017

Hill, M. N., Ho, W. S., Sinopoli, K. J., Viau, V., Hillard, C. J., & Gorzalka, B. B. (2006). Involvement of the endocannabinoid system in the ability of long-term tricyclic antidepressant treatment to suppress stress-induced activation of the hypothalamic-pituitary-adrenal axis. *Neuropsychopharmacology : official publication of the American College of Neuropsychopharmacology, 31*(12), 2591–2599. https://doi.org/10.1038/sj.npp.1301092

Hill, M. N., Patel, S., Campolongo, P., Tasker, J. G., Wotjak, C. T., & Bains, J. S. (2010). Functional interactions between stress and the endocannabinoid system: from synaptic signaling to behavioral output. *The Journal of neuroscience : the official journal of the Society for Neuroscience, 30*(45), 14980–14986. https://doi.org/10.1523/JNEUROSCI.4283-10.2010

Hill, T. D., Cascio, M. G., Romano, B., Duncan, M., Pertwee, R. G., Williams, C. M., Whalley, B. J., & Hill, A. J. (2013). Cannabidivarin-rich cannabis extracts are anticonvulsant in mouse and rat via a CB1 receptor-independent mechanism. *British journal of pharmacology, 170*(3), 679–692. https://doi.org/10.1111/bph.12321

Hirvonen, J., Goodwin, R. S., Li, C. T., Terry, G. E., Zoghbi, S. S., Morse, C., Pike, V. W., Volkow, N. D., Huestis, M. A., & Innis, R. B. (2012). Reversible and regionally selective downregulation of brain cannabinoid CB1 receptors in chronic daily cannabis smokers. *Molecular psychiatry*, 17(6), 642– 649. https://doi.org/10.1038/mp.2011.82

Hossain, K. R., Alghalayini, A., & Valenzuela, S. M. (2023). Current Challenges and Opportunities for Improved Cannabidiol Solubility. *International journal of molecular sciences*, 24(19), 14514. https://doi.org/10.3390/ijms241914514

Hsiao, E. Y., McBride, S. W., Hsien, S., Sharon, G., Hyde, E. R., McCue, T., Codelli, J. A., Chow, J., Reisman, S. E., Petrosino, J. F., Patterson, P. H., & Mazmanian, S. K. (2013). Microbiota modulate behavioral and physiological abnormalities associated with neurodevelopmental disorders. *Cell*, 155(7), 1451–1463. https://doi.org/10.1016/j.cell.2013.11.024

Hsu, S. S., Huang, C. J., Cheng, H. H., Chou, C. T., Lee, H. Y., Wang, J. L., Chen, I. S., Liu, S. I., Lu, Y. C., Chang, H. T., Huang, J. K., Chen, J. S., & Jan, C. R. (2007). Anandamide-induced Ca2+ elevation leading to p38 MAPK phosphorylation and subsequent cell death via apoptosis in human osteosarcoma cells. *Toxicology*, 231(1), 21–29. https://doi.org/10.1016/j.tox.2006.11.005

Huang, J. Y., Fang, M., Li, Y. J., Ma, Y. Q., & Cai, X. H. (2010). *Nan fang yi ke da xue xue bao = Journal of Southern Medical University*, 30(9), 2161–2164.

Hu, J., Zhang, J., Hu, L., Yu, H., & Xu, J. (2021). Art Therapy: A Complementary Treatment for Mental Disorders. *Frontiers in psychology*, 12, 686005. https://doi.org/10.3389/fpsyg.2021.686005

Hutchins-Wiese, H. L., Li, Y., Hannon, K., & Watkins, B. A. (2012). Hind limb suspension and long-chain omega-3 PUFA increase mRNA endocannabinoid system levels in skeletal muscle. *The Journal of nutritional biochemistry*, 23(8), 986–993. https://doi.org/10.1016/j.jnutbio.2011.05.005

Hutten, N. R. P. W., Arkell, T. R., Vinckenbosch, F., Schepers, J., Kevin, R. C., Theunissen, E. L., Kuypers, K. P. C., McGregor, I. S., & Ramaekers, J. G. (2022). Cannabis containing equivalent concentrations of delta-9-tetrahydrocannabinol (THC) and cannabidiol (CBD) induces less state anxiety than THC-dominant cannabis. *Psychopharmacology*, 239(11), 3731–3741. https://doi.org/10.1007/s00213-022-06248-9

Iden, J. A., Raphael-Mizrahi, B., Awida, Z., Naim, A., Zyc, D., Liron, T., Kasher, M., Livshits, G., Vered, M., & Gabet, Y. (2023). The Anti-Tumorigenic Role of Cannabinoid Receptor 2 in Colon Cancer: A Study in Mice and Humans. *International journal of molecular sciences*, 24(4), 4060. https://doi.org/10.3390/ijms24044060

Innes, J. K., & Calder, P. C. (2018). Omega-6 fatty acids and inflammation. *Prostaglandins, leukotrienes, and essential fatty acids*, 132, 41–48. https://doi.org/10.1016/j.plefa.2018.03.004

Izzo, A. A., Fezza, F., Capasso, R., Bisogno, T., Pinto, L., Iuvone, T., Esposito, G., Mascolo, N., Di Marzo, V., & Capasso, F. (2001). Cannabinoid CB1-receptor mediated regulation of gastrointestinal motility in mice in a model of intestinal inflammation. *British journal of pharmacology*, 134(3), 563–570. https://doi.org/10.1038/sj.bjp.0704293

Izzo, A. A., Aviello, G., Petrosino, S., Orlando, P., Marsicano, G., Lutz, B., Borrelli, F., Capasso, R., Nigam, S., Capasso, F., Di Marzo, V., & Endocannabinoid Research Group (2008). Increased endocannabinoid levels reduce the development of precancerous lesions in the mouse colon. *Journal of molecular medicine (Berlin, Germany)*, 86(1), 89–98. https://doi.org/10.1007/s00109-007-0248-4

Jackson, S. J., Pryce, G., Diemel, L. T., Cuzner, M. L., & Baker, D. (2005). Cannabinoid-receptor 1 null mice are susceptible to neurofilament damage and caspase 3 activation. *Neuroscience*, 134(1), 261– 268. https://doi.org/10.1016/j.neuroscience.2005.02.045

Jamil, A., Gutlapalli, S. D., Ali, M., Oble, M. J. P., Sonia, S. N., George, S., Shahi, S. R., Ali, Z., Abaza, A., & Mohammed, L. (2023). Meditation and Its Mental and Physical Health Benefits in 2023. *Cureus*, 15(6), e40650. https://doi.org/10.7759/cureus.40650

Jansma, J., Brinkman, F., van Hemert, S., & El Aidy, S. (2021). Targeting the endocannabinoid system with microbial interventions to improve gut integrity. *Progress in neuro-psychopharmacology & biological psychiatry*, 106, 110169. https://doi.org/10.1016/j.pnpbp.2020.110169

Jin P. (1992). Efficacy of Tai Chi, brisk walking, meditation, and reading in reducing mental and emotional stress. *Journal of psychosomatic research*, 36(4), 361–370. https://doi.org/10.1016/0022-3999(92)90072-a

Jonsson, K. O., Vandevoorde, S., Lambert, D. M., Tiger, G., & Fowler, C. J. (2001). Effects of homologues and analogues of palmitoylethanolamide upon the inactivation of the endocannabinoid anandamide. *British journal of pharmacology*, 133(8), 1263–1275. https://doi.org/10.1038/sj.bjp.0704199

Julien, B., Grenard, P., Teixeira-Clerc, F., Van Nhieu, J. T., Li, L., Karsak, M., Zimmer, A., Mallat, A., & Lotersztajn, S. (2005). Antifibrogenic role of the cannabinoid receptor CB2 in the liver. *Gastroenterology*, 128(3), 742–755. https://doi.org/10.1053/j.gastro.2004.12.050

Kaliman, P., Alvarez-López, M. J., Cosín-Tomás, M., Rosenkranz, M. A., Lutz, A., & Davidson, R. J. (2014). Rapid changes in histone deacetylases and inflammatory gene expression in expert meditators. *Psychoneuroendocrinology*, 40, 96–107. https://doi.org/10.1016/j.psyneuen.2013.11.004

Kenyon, J., Liu, W., & Dalgleish, A. (2018). Report of Objective Clinical Responses of Cancer Patients to Pharmaceutical-grade Synthetic Cannabidiol. *Anticancer research*, 38(10), 5831–5835. https://doi.org/10.21873/anticanres.12924

Keir S. T. (2011). Effect of massage therapy on stress levels and quality of life in brain tumor patients-- observations from a pilot study. *Supportive care in cancer : official journal of the Multinational Association of Supportive Care in Cancer*, 19(5), 711–715. https://doi.org/10.1007/s00520-010-1032-5

Khan, S. U., Lone, A. N., Khan, M. S., Virani, S. S., Blumenthal, R. S., Nasir, K., Miller, M., Michos, E. D., Ballantyne, C. M., Boden, W. E., & Bhatt, D. L. (2021). Effect of omega-3 fatty acids on cardiovascular outcomes: A systematic review and meta-analysis. *EClinicalMedicine*, 38, 100997. https://doi.org/10.1016/j.eclinm.2021.100997

Kiecolt-Glaser J. K. (2010). Stress, food, and inflammation: psychoneuroimmunology and nutrition at the cutting edge. *Psychosomatic medicine*, 72(4), 365–369.https://doi.org/10.1097/PSY.0b013e3181dbf489

Kiecolt-Glaser, J. K., Belury, M. A., Porter, K., Beversdorf, D. Q., Lemeshow, S., & Glaser, R. (2007). Depressive symptoms, omega-6:omega-3 fatty acids, and inflammation in older adults. *Psychosomatic medicine*, 69(3), 217–224. https://doi.org/10.1097/PSY.0b013e3180313a45

Kim, I. B., & Park, S. C. (2021). The Entorhinal Cortex and Adult Neurogenesis in Major Depression. *International journal of molecular sciences*, 22(21), 11725. https://doi.org/10.3390/ijms222111725

Kim, S. D. (2014). Effects of yogic exercises on life stress and blood glucose levels in nursing students. *Journal of physical therapy science*, 26(12), 2003–2006. https://doi.org/10.1589/jpts.26.2003

King, A. R., Dotsey, E. Y., Lodola, A., Jung, K. M., Ghomian, A., Qiu, Y., Fu, J., Mor, M., & Piomelli, D. (2009). Discovery of potent and reversible monoacylglycerol lipase inhibitors. *Chemistry & biology*, 16(10), 1045–1052. https://doi.org/10.1016/j.chembiol.2009.09.012

Kitajima, M., Iwai, M., Kikura-Hanajiri, R., Goda, Y., Iida, M., Yabushita, H., & Takayama, H. (2011). Discovery of indole alkaloids with cannabinoid CB1 receptor antagonistic activity. *Bioorganic & medicinal chemistry letters*, 21(7), 1962–1964. https://doi.org/10.1016/j.bmcl.2011.02.036

Kober, A. K. M. H., Saha, S., Ayyash, M., Namai, F., Nishiyama, K., Yoda, K., Villena, J., & Kitazawa, H. (2024). Insights into the Anti-Adipogenic and Anti-Inflammatory Potentialities of Probiotics against Obesity. *Nutrients*, 16(9), 1373. https://doi.org/10.3390/nu16091373

Koch M. (2017). Cannabinoid Receptor Signaling in Central Regulation of Feeding Behavior: A Mini- Review. *Frontiers in neuroscience*, 11, 293. https://doi.org/10.3389/fnins.2017.00293

Kopsky, D. J., & Hesselink, J. M. (2012). Multimodal stepped care approach with acupuncture and PPAR-α agonist palmitoylethanolamide in the treatment of a patient with multiple sclerosis and central neuropathic pain. *Acupuncture in medicine : journal of the British Medical Acupuncture Society*, 30(1), 53–55. https://doi.org/10.1136/acupmed-2011-010119

Korte, G., Dreiseitel, A., Schreier, P., Oehme, A., Locher, S., Geiger, S., Heilmann, J., & Sand, P. G. (2010). Tea catechins' affinity for human cannabinoid receptors. *Phytomedicine : international journal of phytotherapy and phytopharmacology*, 17(1), 19–22. https://doi.org/10.1016/j.phymed.2009.10.001

Korte, G., Dreiseitel, A., Schreier, P., Oehme, A., Locher, S., Hajak, G., & Sand, P. G. (2009). An examination of anthocyanins' and anthocyanidins' affinity for cannabinoid receptors. *Journal of medicinal food, 12*(6), 1407–1410. https://doi.org/10.1089/jmf.2008.0243

Kostoglou-Athanassiou, I., Athanassiou, L., & Athanassiou, P. (2020). The Effect of Omega-3 Fatty Acids on Rheumatoid Arthritis. *Mediterranean journal of rheumatology, 31*(2), 190–194. https://doi.org/10.31138/mjr.31.2.190

Kroon, E., Kuhns, L., Hoch, E., & Cousijn, J. (2020). Heavy cannabis use, dependence and the brain: a clinical perspective. *Addiction (Abingdon, England), 115*(3), 559–572. https://doi.org/10.1111/add.14776

Kvist, K., Laursen, A. S. D., Overvad, K., & Jakobsen, M. U. (2020). Substitution of Milk with Whole-Fat Yogurt Products or Cheese Is Associated with a Lower Risk of Myocardial Infarction: The Danish Diet, Cancer and Health cohort. *The Journal of nutrition, 150*(5), 1252–1258. https://doi.org/10.1093/jn/nxz337

Lafourcade, M., Larrieu, T., Mato, S., Duffaud, A., Sepers, M., Matias, I., De Smedt-Peyrusse, V., Labrousse, V. F., Bretillon, L., Matute, C., Rodríguez-Puertas, R., Layé, S., & Manzoni, O. J. (2011). Nutritional omega-3 deficiency abolishes endocannabinoid-mediated neuronal functions. *Nature neuroscience, 14*(3), 345–350. https://doi.org/10.1038/nn.2736

Laine, K., Järvinen, K., & Järvinen, T. (2003). Topically administered CB(2)-receptor agonist, JWH-133, does not decrease intraocular pressure (IOP) in normotensive rabbits. *Life sciences, 72*(7), 837– 842. https://doi.org/10.1016/s0024-3205(02)02339-1

Lake, K. D., Martin, B. R., Kunos, G., & Varga, K. (1997). Cardiovascular effects of anandamide in anesthetized and conscious normotensive and hypertensive rats. *Hypertension (Dallas, Tex. : 1979), 29*(5), 1204–1210. https://doi.org/10.1161/01.hyp.29.5.1204

Lastres-Becker, I., Cebeira, M., de Ceballos, M. L., Zeng, B. Y., Jenner, P., Ramos, J. A., & Fernández-Ruiz, J. J. (2001). Increased cannabinoid CB1 receptor binding and activation of GTP-binding proteins in the basal ganglia of patients with Parkinson's syndrome and of MPTP-treated marmosets. *The European journal of neuroscience, 14*(11), 1827–1832. https://doi.org/10.1046/j.0953- 816x.2001.01812.x

Laviolette, S. R., & Grace, A. A. (2006). The roles of cannabinoid and dopamine receptor systems in neural emotional learning circuits: implications for schizophrenia and addiction. *Cellular and molecular life sciences : CMLS, 63*(14), 1597–1613. https://doi.org/10.1007/s00018-006-6027-5

Lazar, S. W., Kerr, C. E., Wasserman, R. H., Gray, J. R., Greve, D. N., Treadway, M. T., McGarvey, M., Quinn, B. T., Dusek, J. A., Benson, H., Rauch, S. L., Moore, C. I., & Fischl, B. (2005). Meditation experience is associated with increased cortical thickness. *Neuroreport, 16*(17), 1893–1897. https://doi.org/10.1097/01.wnr.0000186598.66243.19

León, F., Gao, J., Dale, O. R., Wu, Y., Habib, E., Husni, A. S., Hill, R. A., & Cutler, S. J. (2013). Secondary metabolites from Eupenicillium parvum and their in vitro binding affinity for human opioid and cannabinoid receptors. *Planta medica, 79*(18), 1756–1761. https://doi.org/10.1055/s-0033-1351099

Leonti, M., Casu, L., Raduner, S., Cottiglia, F., Floris, C., Altmann, K. H., & Gertsch, J. (2010). Falcarinol is a covalent cannabinoid CB1 receptor antagonist and induces pro-allergic effects in skin. *Biochemical pharmacology, 79*(12), 1815–1826. https://doi.org/10.1016/j.bcp.2010.02.015

Le Strat, Y., & Le Foll, B. (2011). Obesity and cannabis use: results from 2 representative national surveys. *American journal of epidemiology, 174*(8), 929–933. https://doi.org/10.1093/aje/kwr200

Leweke, F. M., Piomelli, D., Pahlisch, F., Muhl, D., Gerth, C. W., Hoyer, C., Klosterkötter, J., Hellmich, M., & Koethe, D. (2012). Cannabidiol enhances anandamide signaling and alleviates psychotic symptoms of schizophrenia. *Translational psychiatry, 2*(3), e94. https://doi.org/10.1038/tp.2012.15

Lewis, D. A., Hashimoto, T., & Volk, D. W. (2005). Cortical inhibitory neurons and schizophrenia. *Nature reviews. Neuroscience, 6*(4), 312–324. https://doi.org/10.1038/nrn1648

Liang, C., McClean, M. D., Marsit, C., Christensen, B., Peters, E., Nelson, H. H., & Kelsey, K. T. (2009). A population-based case-control study of marijuana use and head and neck squamous cell carcinoma. *Cancer prevention research (Philadelphia, Pa.), 2*(8), 759–768. https://doi.org/10.1158/1940-6207.CAPR-09-0048

Ligresti, A., Villano, R., Allarà, M., Ujváry, I., & Di Marzo, V. (2012). Kavalactones and the endocannabinoid system: the plant-derived yangonin is a novel CB₁ receptor ligand. *Pharmacological research*, 66(2), 163–169. https://doi.org/10.1016/j.phrs.2012.04.003

Lim, H. K., Lee, H. R., & Do, S. H. (2015). Stimulation of cannabinoid receptors by using Rubus coreanus extracts to control osteoporosis in aged male rats. *The aging male : the official journal of the International Society for the Study of the Aging Male*, 18(2), 124–132. https://doi.org/10.3109/13685538.2014.949661

Lindgren, L., Rundgren, S., Winsö, O., Lehtipalo, S., Wiklund, U., Karlsson, M., Stenlund, H., Jacobsson, C., & Brulin, C. (2010). Physiological responses to touch massage in healthy volunteers. *Autonomic neuroscience : basic & clinical*, 158(1-2), 105–110. https://doi.org/10.1016/j.autneu.2010.06.011

Lindner, T., Schmidl, D., Peschorn, L., Pai, V., Popa-Cherecheanu, A., Chua, J., Schmetterer, L., & Garhöfer, G. (2023). Therapeutic Potential of Cannabinoids in Glaucoma. *Pharmaceuticals (Basel, Switzerland)*, 16(8), 1149. https://doi.org/10.3390/ph16081149

Lin, Y. S., Huang, W. H., Hsu, K. F., Tang, M. J., & Chiu, W. T. (2023). Reversion of chemoresistance by endocannabinoid-induced ER stress and autophagy activation in ovarian cancer. *American journal of cancer research*, 13(9), 4163–4178.

Li, S., Huang, Y., Yu, L., Ji, X., & Wu, J. (2023). Impact of the Cannabinoid System in Alzheimer's Disease. *Current neuropharmacology*, 21(3), 715–726. https://doi.org/10.2174/1570159X20666220201091006

Liu, M. W., Su, M. X., Wang, Y. H., Wei, W., Qin, L. F., Liu, X., Tian, M. L., & Qian, C. Y. (2014). Effect of melilotus extract on lung injury by upregulating the expression of cannabinoid CB2 receptors in septic rats. *BMC complementary and alternative medicine*, 14, 94. https://doi.org/10.1186/1472-6882-14-94

Liu, W. H., Wu, J. S., Hua, L. B., Pan, Z. F., Zhang, H. B., Xu, N. G., & He, Y. H. (2024). Advances in the study of endocannabinoid receptors in experimental acupuncture analgesia. 内源性大麻素受体在针刺镇痛机制中的研究进展. *Zhen ci yan jiu = Acupuncture research*, 49(1), 88–93. https://doi.org/10.13702/j.1000-0607.20230364

Liu, X., Jutooru, I., Lei, P., Kim, K., Lee, S. O., Brents, L. K., Prather, P. L., & Safe, S. (2012). Betulinic acid targets YY1 and ErbB2 through cannabinoid receptor-dependent disruption of microRNA- 27a:ZBTB10 in breast cancer. *Molecular cancer therapeutics*, 11(7), 1421–1431. https://doi.org/10.1158/1535-7163.MCT-12-0026

Long, C., Xie, N., Shu, Y., Wu, Y., He, P., Zhou, Y., Xiang, Y., Gu, J., Yang, L., & Wang, Y. (2021). Knockout of the Cannabinoid Receptor 2 Gene Promotes Inflammation and Hepatic Stellate Cell Activation by Promoting A20/Nuclear Factor-κB (NF-κB) Expression in Mice with Carbon Tetrachloride- Induced Liver Fibrosis. *Medical science monitor : international medical journal of experimental and clinical research*, 27, e931236. https://doi.org/10.12659/MSM.931236

Lopez-Garcia, E., Schulze, M. B., Fung, T. T., Meigs, J. B., Rifai, N., Manson, J. E., & Hu, F. B. (2004). Major dietary patterns are related to plasma concentrations of markers of inflammation and endothelial dysfunction. *The American journal of clinical nutrition*, 80(4), 1029–1035. https://doi.org/10.1093/ajcn/80.4.1029

Lu, H. C., & Mackie, K. (2016). An Introduction to the Endogenous Cannabinoid System. *Biological psychiatry*, 79(7), 516–525. https://doi.org/10.1016/j.biopsych.2015.07.028

Lu, H. C., & Mackie, K. (2021). Review of the Endocannabinoid System. *Biological psychiatry. Cognitive neuroscience and neuroimaging*, 6(6), 607–615. https://doi.org/10.1016/j.bpsc.2020.07.016

Luján, M. Á., & Valverde, O. (2020). The Pro-neurogenic Effects of Cannabidiol and Its Potential Therapeutic Implications in Psychiatric Disorders. *Frontiers in behavioral neuroscience*, 14, 109. https://doi.org/10.3389/fnbeh.2020.00109

Maccarrone, M., Lorenzon, T., Bari, M., Melino, G., & Finazzi-Agro, A. (2000). Anandamide induces apoptosis in human cells via vanilloid receptors. Evidence for a protective role of cannabinoid receptors. *The Journal of biological chemistry*, 275(41), 31938–31945. https://doi.org/10.1074/jbc.M005722200

Mallet, C., Daulhac, L., Bonnefont, J., Ledent, C., Etienne, M., Chapuy, E., Libert, F., & Eschalier, A. (2008). Endocannabinoid and serotonergic systems are needed for acetaminophen-induced analgesia. *Pain*, 139(1), 190–200. https://doi.org/10.1016/j.pain.2008.03.030

Mannekote Thippaiah, S., Iyengar, S. S., & Vinod, K. Y. (2021). Exo- and Endo-cannabinoids in Depressive and Suicidal Behaviors. *Frontiers in psychiatry*, 12, 636228. https://doi.org/10.3389/fpsyt.2021.636228

Manzanares, J., Julian, M., & Carrascosa, A. (2006). Role of the cannabinoid system in pain control and therapeutic implications for the management of acute and chronic pain episodes. *Current neuropharmacology*, 4(3), 239–257. https://doi.org/10.2174/157015906778019527

Marchand W. R. (2012). Mindfulness-based stress reduction, mindfulness-based cognitive therapy, and Zen meditation for depression, anxiety, pain, and psychological distress. *Journal of psychiatric practice*, 18(4), 233–252. https://doi.org/10.1097/01.pra.0000416014.53215.86

Martin, E. I., Ressler, K. J., Binder, E., & Nemeroff, C. B. (2009). The neurobiology of anxiety disorders: brain imaging, genetics, and psychoneuroendocrinology. *The Psychiatric clinics of North America*, 32(3), 549–575. https://doi.org/10.1016/j.psc.2009.05.004

Martinez-Gonzalez, M. A., & Bes-Rastrollo, M. (2014). Dietary patterns, Mediterranean diet, and cardiovascular disease. *Current opinion in lipidology*, 25(1), 20–26. https://doi.org/10.1097/MOL.0000000000000044

Masters, R. C., Liese, A. D., Haffner, S. M., Wagenknecht, L. E., & Hanley, A. J. (2010). Whole and refined grain intakes are related to inflammatory protein concentrations in human plasma. *The Journal of nutrition*, 140(3), 587–594. https://doi.org/10.3945/jn.109.116640

Matei, D., Trofin, D., Iordan, D. A., Onu, I., Condurache, I., Ionite, C., & Buculei, I. (2023). The Endocannabinoid System and Physical Exercise. *International journal of molecular sciences*, 24(3), 1989. https://doi.org/10.3390/ijms24031989

McHugh, D., Hu, S. S., Rimmerman, N., Juknat, A., Vogel, Z., Walker, J. M., & Bradshaw, H. B. (2010). N-arachidonoyl glycine, an abundant endogenous lipid, potently drives directed cellular migration through GPR18, the putative abnormal cannabidiol receptor. *BMC neuroscience*, 11, 44. https://doi.org/10.1186/1471-2202-11-44

McPartland, J. M., Giuffrida, A., King, J., Skinner, E., Scotter, J., & Musty, R. E. (2005). Cannabimimetic effects of osteopathic manipulative treatment. *The Journal of the American Osteopathic Association*, 105(6), 283–291.

McPartland J. M. (2008). The endocannabinoid system: an osteopathic perspective. *The Journal of the American Osteopathic Association*, 108(10), 586–600. https://doi.org/10.7556/jaoa.2008.108.10.586

Meschler, J. P., & Howlett, A. C. (1999). Thujone exhibits low affinity for cannabinoid receptors but fails to evoke cannabimimetic responses. *Pharmacology, biochemistry, and behavior*, 62(3), 473–480. https://doi.org/10.1016/s0091-3057(98)00195-6

Michalski, C. W., Oti, F. E., Erkan, M., Sauliunaite, D., Bergmann, F., Pacher, P., Batkai, S., Müller, M. W., Giese, N. A., Friess, H., & Kleeff, J. (2008). Cannabinoids in pancreatic cancer: correlation with survival and pain. *International journal of cancer*, 122(4), 742–750. https://doi.org/10.1002/ijc.23114

Miller, P., Lawrie, S. M., Hodges, A., Clafferty, R., Cosway, R., & Johnstone, E. C. (2001). Genetic liability, illicit drug use, life stress and psychotic symptoms: preliminary findings from the Edinburgh study of people at high risk for schizophrenia. *Social psychiatry and psychiatric epidemiology*, 36(7), 338–342. https://doi.org/10.1007/s001270170038

Miller, S., Daily, L., Leishman, E., Bradshaw, H., & Straiker, A. (2018). Δ9-Tetrahydrocannabinol and Cannabidiol Differentially Regulate Intraocular Pressure. *Investigative ophthalmology & visual science*, 59(15), 5904–5911. https://doi.org/10.1167/iovs.18-24838

Milligan, A. L., Szabo-Pardi, T. A., & Burton, M. D. (2020). Cannabinoid Receptor Type 1 and Its Role as an Analgesic: An Opioid Alternative?. *Journal of dual diagnosis*, 16(1), 106–119. https://doi.org/10.1080/15504263.2019.1668100

Milton N. G. (2002). Anandamide and noladin ether prevent neurotoxicity of the human amyloid-beta peptide. *Neuroscience letters*, 332(2), 127–130. https://doi.org/10.1016/s0304-3940(02)00936-9

Mimeault, M., Pommery, N., Wattez, N., Bailly, C., & Hénichart, J. P. (2003). Anti-proliferative and apoptotic effects of anandamide in human prostatic cancer cell lines: implication of epidermal growth factor receptor down-regulation and ceramide production. *The Prostate*, 56(1), 1–12. https://doi.org/10.1002/pros.10190

Mimica, N., & Kalinić, D. (2011). Art therapy may be benefitial for reducing stress--related behaviours in people with dementia--case report. *Psychiatria Danubina*, 23(1), 125–128. Montaser, R., Paul, V. J., & Luesch, H. (2012). Marine cyanobacterial fatty acid amides acting on cannabinoid receptors. *Chembiochem : a European journal of chemical biology*, 13(18), 2676– 2681. https://doi.org/10.1002/cbic.201200502

More, S. V., & Choi, D. K. (2015). Promising cannabinoid-based therapies for Parkinson's disease: motor symptoms to neuroprotection. *Molecular neurodegeneration*, 10, 17. https://doi.org/10.1186/s13024-015-0012-0

Muccioli, G. G., Naslain, D., Bäckhed, F., Reigstad, C. S., Lambert, D. M., Delzenne, N. M., & Cani, P. D. (2010). The endocannabinoid system links gut microbiota to adipogenesis. *Molecular systems biology*, 6, 392. https://doi.org/10.1038/msb.2010.46

Naftali, T., Bar-Lev Schleider, L., Dotan, I., Lansky, E. P., Sklerovsky Benjaminov, F., & Konikoff, F. M. (2013). Cannabis induces a clinical response in patients with Crohn's disease: a prospective placebo-controlled study. *Clinical gastroenterology and hepatology : the official clinical practice journal of the American Gastroenterological Association*, 11(10), 1276–1280.e1. https://doi.org/10.1016/j.cgh.2013.04.034

Nahler G. (2022). Cannabidiol and Other Phytocannabinoids as Cancer Therapeutics. *Pharmaceutical medicine*, 36(2), 99–129. https://doi.org/10.1007/s40290-022-00420-4

Nakane, S., Tanaka, T., Satouchi, K., Kobayashi, Y., Waku, K., & Sugiura, T. (2000). Occurrence of a novel cannabimimetic molecule 2-sciadonoylglycerol (2-eicosa-5',11',14'-trienoylglycerol) in the umbrella pine Sciadopitys verticillata seeds. *Biological & pharmaceutical bulletin*, 23(6), 758– 761. https://doi.org/10.1248/bpb.23.758

Negus S. S. (2006). Some implications of receptor theory for in vivo assessment of agonists, antagonists and inverse agonists. *Biochemical pharmacology*, 71(12), 1663–1670. https://doi.org/10.1016/j.bcp.2005.12.038

Nehlig A. (2013). The neuroprotective effects of cocoa flavanol and its influence on cognitive performance. *British journal of clinical pharmacology*, 75(3), 716–727. https://doi.org/10.1111/j.1365-2125.2012.04378.x

Neuschwander-Tetri B. A. (2007). Food energy efficiency, cannabinoids, and a slow death of the weight loss dogma. *Hepatology (Baltimore, Md.)*, 46(1), 12–15. https://doi.org/10.1002/hep.21821

Newell, K. A., Deng, C., & Huang, X. F. (2006). Increased cannabinoid receptor density in the posterior cingulate cortex in schizophrenia. *Experimental brain research*, 172(4), 556–560. https://doi.org/10.1007/s00221-006-0503-x

Nguyen, B. M., Kim, D., Bricker, S., Bongard, F., Neville, A., Putnam, B., Smith, J., & Plurad, D. (2014). Effect of marijuana use on outcomes in traumatic brain injury. *The American surgeon*, 80(10), 979–983.

Nicolussi, S., Viveros-Paredes, J. M., Gachet, M. S., Rau, M., Flores-Soto, M. E., Blunder, M., & Gertsch, J. (2014). Guineensine is a novel inhibitor of endocannabinoid uptake showing cannabimimetic behavioral effects in BALB/c mice. *Pharmacological research*, 80, 52–65.https://doi.org/10.1016/j.phrs.2013.12.010

Oh, J. H., Kang, L. L., Ban, J. O., Kim, Y. H., Kim, K. H., Han, S. B., & Hong, J. T. (2009). Anti-inflammatory effect of 4-O-methylhonokiol, compound isolated from Magnolia officinalis through inhibition of NF-kappaB [corrected]. *Chemico-biological interactions*, 180(3), 506–514. https://doi.org/10.1016/j.cbi.2009.03.014

Oliveira, C. D. C., Castor, M. G. M. E., Castor, C. G. M. E., Costa, Á. F., Ferreira, R. C. M., Silva, J. F. D., Pelaez, J. M. N., Capettini, L. D. S. A., Lemos, V. S., Duarte, I. D. G., Perez, A. C., Santos, S. H. S., & Romero, T. R. L. (2019). Evidence for the involvement of opioid and cannabinoid systems in the peripheral antinociception mediated by resveratrol. *Toxicology and applied pharmacology*, 369, 30–38. https://doi.org/10.1016/j.taap.2019.02.004

Oliveira, N. M. C., Machado, D. A., da Silva, T. L., & do Vale, G. T. (2022). Treatment with Cannabidiol Results in an Antioxidant and Cardioprotective Effect in Several Pathophysiologies. *Current hypertension reviews*, 18(2), 125–129. https://doi.org/10.2174/1573402118666220513164101

O'Sullivan S. E. (2007). Cannabinoids go nuclear: evidence for activation of peroxisome proliferator- activated receptors. *British journal of pharmacology*, 152(5), 576–582. https://doi.org/10.1038/sj.bjp.0707423

O'Sullivan, S. E., Yates, A. S., & Porter, R. K. (2021). The Peripheral Cannabinoid Receptor Type 1 (CB$_1$) as a Molecular Target for Modulating Body Weight in Man. *Molecules (Basel, Switzerland)*, 26(20), 6178. https://doi.org/10.3390/molecules26206178

Oteng, A. B., & Kersten, S. (2020). Mechanisms of Action of trans Fatty Acids. *Advances in nutrition (Bethesda, Md.)*, 11(3), 697–708. https://doi.org/10.1093/advances/nmz125

Otto, T., & Sicinski, P. (2017). Cell cycle proteins as promising targets in cancer therapy. *Nature reviews. Cancer*, 17(2), 93–115. https://doi.org/10.1038/nrc.2016.138

Overton, H. A., Fyfe, M. C., & Reynet, C. (2008). GPR119, a novel G protein-coupled receptor target for the treatment of type 2 diabetes and obesity. *British journal of pharmacology*, 153 Suppl 1(Suppl 1), S76–S81. https://doi.org/10.1038/sj.bjp.0707529

Pacher, P., Bátkai, S., & Kunos, G. (2006). The endocannabinoid system as an emerging target of pharmacotherapy. *Pharmacological reviews*, 58(3), 389–462. https://doi.org/10.1124/pr.58.3.2

Pacher, P., & Kunos, G. (2013). Modulating the endocannabinoid system in human health and disease-- successes and failures. *The FEBS journal*, 280(9), 1918–1943. https://doi.org/10.1111/febs.12260

Paland, N., Hamza, H., Pechkovsky, A., Aswad, M., Shagidov, D., & Louria-Hayon, I. (2023). Cannabis and Rheumatoid Arthritis: A Scoping Review Evaluating the Benefits, Risks, and Future Research Directions. *Rambam Maimonides medical journal*, 14(4), e0022. https://doi.org/10.5041/RMMJ.10509

Palermo, F. A., Mosconi, G., Avella, M. A., Carnevali, O., Verdenelli, M. C., Cecchini, C., & Polzonetti- Magni, A. M. (2011). Modulation of cortisol levels, endocannabinoid receptor 1A, proopiomelanocortin and thyroid hormone receptor alpha mRNA expressions by probiotics during sole (Solea solea) larval development. *General and comparative endocrinology*, 171(3), 293–300. https://doi.org/10.1016/j.ygcen.2011.02.009

Palu, A. K., Kim, A. H., West, B. J., Deng, S., Jensen, J., & White, L. (2008). The effects of Morinda citrifolia L. (noni) on the immune system: its molecular mechanisms of action. *Journal of ethnopharmacology*, 115(3), 502–506. https://doi.org/10.1016/j.jep.2007.10.023

Pandey, R., Mousawy, K., Nagarkatti, M., & Nagarkatti, P. (2009). Endocannabinoids and immune regulation. *Pharmacological research*, 60(2), 85–92. https://doi.org/10.1016/j.phrs.2009.03.019

Papier, K., Hartman, L., Tong, T. Y. N., Key, T. J., & Knuppel, A. (2022). Higher Meat Intake Is Associated with Higher Inflammatory Markers, Mostly Due to Adiposity: Results from UK Biobank. *The Journal of nutrition*, 152(1), 183–189. https://doi.org/10.1093/jn/nxab314

Park, M., Lee, J. H., Choi, J. K., Hong, Y. D., Bae, I. H., Lim, K. M., Park, Y. H., & Ha, H. (2014). 18β- glycyrrhetinic acid attenuates anandamide-induced adiposity and high-fat diet induced obesity. *Molecular nutrition & food research*, 58(7), 1436–1446. https://doi.org/10.1002/mnfr.201300763

Patel, S., & Hillard, C. J. (2009). Role of endocannabinoid signaling in anxiety and depression. *Current topics in behavioral neurosciences*, 1, 347–371. https://doi.org/10.1007/978-3-540-88955-7_14

Patsos, H. A., Greenhough, A., Hicks, D. J., Al Kharusi, M., Collard, T. J., Lane, J. D., Paraskeva, C., & Williams, A. C. (2010). The endogenous cannabinoid, anandamide, induces COX-2-dependent cell death in apoptosis-resistant colon cancer cells. *International journal of oncology*, 37(1), 187–193. https://doi.org/10.3892/ijo_00000666

Penner, E. A., Buettner, H., & Mittleman, M. A. (2013). The impact of marijuana use on glucose, insulin, and insulin resistance among US adults. *The American journal of medicine*, 126(7), 583–589. https://doi.org/10.1016/j.amjmed.2013.03.002

Pereira, A., Pfeifer, T. A., Grigliatti, T. A., & Andersen, R. J. (2009). Functional cell-based screening and saturation transfer double-difference NMR have identified haplosamate A as a cannabinoid receptor agonist. *ACS chemical biology*, 4(2), 139–144. https://doi.org/10.1021/cb800264k

Pertwee R. G. (2001). Cannabinoids and the gastrointestinal tract. *Gut*, 48(6), 859–867. https://doi.org/10.1136/gut.48.6.859

Pertwee R. G. (2008). The diverse CB1 and CB2 receptor pharmacology of three plant cannabinoids: delta9-tetrahydrocannabinol, cannabidiol and delta9-tetrahydrocannabivarin. *British journal of pharmacology*, 153(2), 199–215. https://doi.org/10.1038/sj.bjp.0707442

Piñeiro, R., & Falasca, M. (2012). Lysophosphatidylinositol signalling: new wine from an old bottle. *Biochimica et biophysica acta*, 1821(4), 694–705. https://doi.org/10.1016/j.bbalip.2012.01.009

Pistis, M., Perra, S., Pillolla, G., Melis, M., Gessa, G. L., & Muntoni, A. L. (2004). Cannabinoids modulate neuronal firing in the rat basolateral amygdala: evidence for CB1- and non-CB1-mediated actions. *Neuropharmacology, 46*(1), 115–125. https://doi.org/10.1016/j.neuropharm.2003.08.003

Porcella, A., Maxia, C., Gessa, G. L., & Pani, L. (2000). The human eye expresses high levels of CB1 cannabinoid receptor mRNA and protein. *The European journal of neuroscience, 12*(3), 1123– 1127. https://doi.org/10.1046/j.1460-9568.2000.01027.x

Pryce, G., Ahmed, Z., Hankey, D. J., Jackson, S. J., Croxford, J. L., Pocock, J. M., Ledent, C., Petzold, A., Thompson, A. J., Giovannoni, G., Cuzner, M. L., & Baker, D. (2003). Cannabinoids inhibit neurodegeneration in models of multiple sclerosis. *Brain : a journal of neurology, 126*(Pt 10), 2191–2202. https://doi.org/10.1093/brain/awg224

Pryce, G., & Baker, D. (2007). Control of spasticity in a multiple sclerosis model is mediated by CB1, not CB2, cannabinoid receptors. *British journal of pharmacology, 150*(4), 519–525. https://doi.org/10.1038/sj.bjp.0707003

Quistad, G. B., Sparks, S. E., & Casida, J. E. (2001). Fatty acid amide hydrolase inhibition by neurotoxic organophosphorus pesticides. *Toxicology and applied pharmacology, 173*(1), 48–55. https://doi.org/10.1006/taap.2001.9175

Rajesh, M., Mukhopadhyay, P., Bátkai, S., Patel, V., Saito, K., Matsumoto, S., Kashiwaya, Y., Horváth, B., Mukhopadhyay, B., Becker, L., Haskó, G., Liaudet, L., Wink, D. A., Veves, A., Mechoulam, R., & Pacher, P. (2010). Cannabidiol attenuates cardiac dysfunction, oxidative stress, fibrosis, and inflammatory and cell death signaling pathways in diabetic cardiomyopathy. *Journal of the American College of Cardiology, 56*(25), 2115–2125. https://doi.org/10.1016/j.jacc.2010.07.033

Rajmohan, R., & Reddy, P. H. (2017). Amyloid-Beta and Phosphorylated Tau Accumulations Cause Abnormalities at Synapses of Alzheimer's disease Neurons. *Journal of Alzheimer's disease : JAD, 57*(4), 975–999. https://doi.org/10.3233/JAD-160612

Raman, C., McAllister, S. D., Rizvi, G., Patel, S. G., Moore, D. H., & Abood, M. E. (2004). Amyotrophic lateral sclerosis: delayed disease progression in mice by treatment with a cannabinoid. *Amyotrophic lateral sclerosis and other motor neuron disorders : official publication of the World Federation of Neurology, Research Group on Motor Neuron Diseases, 5*(1), 33–39. https://doi.org/10.1080/14660820310016813

Ramírez, B. G., Blázquez, C., Gómez del Pulgar, T., Guzmán, M., & de Ceballos, M. L. (2005). Prevention of Alzheimer's disease pathology by cannabinoids: neuroprotection mediated by blockade of microglial activation. *The Journal of neuroscience : the official journal of the Society for Neuroscience, 25*(8), 1904–1913. https://doi.org/10.1523/JNEUROSCI.4540-04.2005

Ramos, J. A., & Bianco, F. J. (2012). The role of cannabinoids in prostate cancer: Basic science perspective and potential clinical applications. *Indian journal of urology : IJU : journal of the Urological Society of India, 28*(1), 9–14. https://doi.org/10.4103/0970-1591.94942

Ravi, J., Sneh, A., Shilo, K., Nasser, M. W., & Ganju, R. K. (2014). FAAH inhibition enhances anandamide mediated anti-tumorigenic effects in non-small cell lung cancer by downregulating the EGF/EGFR pathway. *Oncotarget, 5*(9), 2475–2486. https://doi.org/10.18632/oncotarget.1723

Rempel, V., Fuchs, A., Hinz, S., Karcz, T., Lehr, M., Koetter, U., & Müller, C. E. (2012). Magnolia Extract, Magnolol, and Metabolites: Activation of Cannabinoid CB2 Receptors and Blockade of the Related GPR55. *ACS medicinal chemistry letters, 4*(1), 41–45. https://doi.org/10.1021/ml300235q

Rey, A. A., Purrio, M., Viveros, M. P., & Lutz, B. (2012). Biphasic effects of cannabinoids in anxiety responses: CB1 and GABA(B) receptors in the balance of GABAergic and glutamatergic neurotransmission. *Neuropsychopharmacology : official publication of the American College of Neuropsychopharmacology, 37*(12), 2624–2634. https://doi.org/10.1038/npp.2012.123

Riebe, C. J., & Wotjak, C. T. (2011). Endocannabinoids and stress. *Stress (Amsterdam, Netherlands), 14*(4), 384–397. https://doi.org/10.3109/10253890.2011.586753

Roberts, A., Harris, K., Outen, B., Bukvic, A., Smith, B., Schultz, A., Bergman, S., & Mondal, D. (2022). Osteopathic Manipulative Medicine: A Brief Review of the Hands-On Treatment Approaches and Their Therapeutic Uses. *Medicines (Basel, Switzerland), 9*(5), 33. https://doi.org/10.3390/medicines9050033

Rog, D. J., Nurmikko, T. J., Friede, T., & Young, C. A. (2005). Randomized, controlled trial of cannabis- based medicine in central pain in multiple sclerosis. *Neurology, 65*(6), 812–819. https://doi.org/10.1212/01.wnl.0000176753.45410.8b

Rollinger, J. M., Schuster, D., Danzl, B., Schwaiger, S., Markt, P., Schmidtke, M., Gertsch, J., Raduner, S., Wolber, G., Langer, T., & Stuppner, H. (2009). In silico target fishing for rationalized ligand discovery exemplified on constituents of Ruta graveolens. Planta medica, 75(3), 195–204. https://doi.org/10.1055/s-0028-1088397

Romero, J., García, L., Fernández-Ruiz, J. J., Cebeira, M., & Ramos, J. A. (1995). Changes in rat brain cannabinoid binding sites after acute and chronic exposure to their endogenous agonist, anandamide, or to delta 9-tetrahydrocannabinol. Pharmacology, biochemistry, and behavior, 51(4), 731–737. https://doi.org/10.1016/0091-3057(95)00023-p

Rousseaux, C., Thuru, X., Gelot, A., Barnich, N., Neut, C., Dubuquoy, L., Dubuquoy, C., Merour, E., Geboes, K., Chamaillard, M., Ouwehand, A., Leyer, G., Carcano, D., Colombel, J. F., Ardid, D., & Desreumaux, P. (2007). Lactobacillus acidophilus modulates intestinal pain and induces opioid and cannabinoid receptors. Nature medicine, 13(1), 35–37. https://doi.org/10.1038/nm1521

Ruegsegger, G. N., & Booth, F. W. (2018). Health Benefits of Exercise. Cold Spring Harbor perspectives in medicine, 8(7), a029694. https://doi.org/10.1101/cshperspect.a029694

Rühl, T., Deuther-Conrad, W., Fischer, S., Günther, R., Hennig, L., Krautscheid, H., & Brust, P. (2012). Cannabinoid receptor type 2 (CB2)-selective N-aryl-oxadiazolyl-propionamides: synthesis, radiolabelling, molecular modelling and biological evaluation. Organic and medicinal chemistry letters, 2(1), 32. https://doi.org/10.1186/2191-2858-2-32

Ruiu, S., Anzani, N., Orrù, A., Floris, C., Caboni, P., Maccioni, E., Distinto, S., Alcaro, S., & Cottiglia, F. (2013). N-Alkyl dien- and trienamides from the roots of Otanthus maritimus with binding affinity for opioid and cannabinoid receptors. Bioorganic & medicinal chemistry, 21(22), 7074– 7082. https://doi.org/10.1016/j.bmc.2013.09.017

Salahudeen, M. S., & Nishtala, P. S. (2017). An overview of pharmacodynamic modelling, ligand-binding approach and its application in clinical practice. Saudi pharmaceutical journal : SPJ : the official publication of the Saudi Pharmaceutical Society, 25(2), 165–175. https://doi.org/10.1016/j.jsps.2016.07.002

Salviato, B. Z., Raymundi, A. M., Rodrigues da Silva, T., Salemme, B. W., Batista Sohn, J. M., Araújo, F. S., Guimarães, F. S., Bertoglio, L. J., & Stern, C. A. (2021). Female but not male rats show biphasic effects of low doses of Δ⁹-tetrahydrocannabinol on anxiety: can cannabidiol interfere with these effects?. Neuropharmacology, 196, 108684. https://doi.org/10.1016/j.neuropharm.2021.108684

Sam, A. H., Salem, V., & Ghatei, M. A. (2011). Rimonabant: From RIO to Ban. Journal of obesity, 2011, 432607. https://doi.org/10.1155/2011/432607

Satokari R. (2020). High Intake of Sugar and the Balance between Pro- and Anti-Inflammatory Gut Bacteria. Nutrients, 12(5), 1348. https://doi.org/10.3390/nu12051348

Schuehly, W., Paredes, J. M., Kleyer, J., Huefner, A., Anavi-Goffer, S., Raduner, S., Altmann, K. H., & Gertsch, J. (2011). Mechanisms of osteoclastogenesis inhibition by a novel class of biphenyl-type cannabinoid CB(2) receptor inverse agonists. Chemistry & biology, 18(8), 1053–1064. https://doi.org/10.1016/j.chembiol.2011.05.012

Schwitzer, T., Schwan, R., Angioi-Duprez, K., Giersch, A., & Laprevote, V. (2016). The Endocannabinoid System in the Retina: From Physiology to Practical and Therapeutic Applications. Neural plasticity, 2016, 2916732. https://doi.org/10.1155/2016/2916732

Sender, R., Fuchs, S., & Milo, R. (2016). Revised Estimates for the Number of Human and Bacteria Cells in the Body. PLoS biology, 14(8), e1002533. https://doi.org/10.1371/journal.pbio.1002533

Seo J. Y. (2009). [The effects of aromatherapy on stress and stress responses in adolescents]. Journal of Korean Academy of Nursing, 39(3), 357–365. https://doi.org/10.4040/jkan.2009.39.3.357

Sharma, C., Sadek, B., Goyal, S. N., Sinha, S., Kamal, M. A., & Ojha, S. (2015). Small Molecules from Nature Targeting G-Protein Coupled Cannabinoid Receptors: Potential Leads for Drug Discovery and Development. Evidence-based complementary and alternative medicine : eCAM, 2015, 238482. https://doi.org/10.1155/2015/238482

Shin, H. S., Ryu, K. H., & Song, Y. A. (2011). [Effects of laughter therapy on postpartum fatigue and stress responses of postpartum women]. Journal of Korean Academy of Nursing, 41(3), 294–301. https://doi.org/10.4040/jkan.2011.41.3.294

Shohami, E., Cohen-Yeshurun, A., Magid, L., Algali, M., & Mechoulam, R. (2011). Endocannabinoids and traumatic brain injury. British journal of pharmacology, 163(7), 1402–1410. https://doi.org/10.1111/j.1476-5381.2011.01343.x

Siebers, M., Biedermann, S. V., Bindila, L., Lutz, B., & Fuss, J. (2021). Exercise-induced euphoria and anxiolysis do not depend on endogenous opioids in humans. *Psychoneuroendocrinology, 126,* 105173. https://doi.org/10.1016/j.psyneuen.2021.105173

Siegmund, S. V., Uchinami, H., Osawa, Y., Brenner, D. A., & Schwabe, R. F. (2005). Anandamide induces necrosis in primary hepatic stellate cells. *Hepatology (Baltimore, Md.), 41*(5), 1085–1095. https://doi.org/10.1002/hep.20667

Simão da Silva, K. A. B., Paszcuk, A. F., Passos, G. F., Silva, E. S., Bento, A. F., Meotti, F. C., & Calixto, J. B. (2011). Activation of cannabinoid receptors by the pentacyclic triterpene α,β-amyrin inhibits inflammatory and neuropathic persistent pain in mice. *Pain, 152*(8), 1872–1887. https://doi.org/10.1016/j.pain.2011.04.005

Simopoulos A. P. (2002). The importance of the ratio of omega-6/omega-3 essential fatty acids. *Biomedicine & pharmacotherapy = Biomedecine & pharmacotherapie, 56*(8), 365–379. https://doi.org/10.1016/s0753-3322(02)00253-6

Singh, Y., & Bali, C. (2013). Cannabis extract treatment for terminal acute lymphoblastic leukemia with a Philadelphia chromosome mutation. *Case reports in oncology, 6*(3), 585–592. https://doi.org/10.1159/000356446

Sinor, A. D., Irvin, S. M., & Greenberg, D. A. (2000). Endocannabinoids protect cerebral cortical neurons from in vitro ischemia in rats. *Neuroscience letters, 278*(3), 157–160. https://doi.org/10.1016/s0304-3940(99)00922-2

Soderstrom, K., Murray, T. F., Yoo, H. D., Ketchum, S., Milligan, K., Gerwick, W., Ortega, M. J., & Salva, J. (1997). Discovery of novel cannabinoid receptor ligands from diverse marine organisms. *Advances in experimental medicine and biology, 433,* 73–77. https://doi.org/10.1007/978-1-4899-1810-9_14

Sofi, F., Macchi, C., Abbate, R., Gensini, G. F., & Casini, A. (2010). Effectiveness of the Mediterranean diet: can it help delay or prevent Alzheimer's disease?. *Journal of Alzheimer's disease : JAD, 20*(3), 795–801. https://doi.org/10.3233/JAD-2010-1418

Soltesz, I., Alger, B. E., Kano, M., Lee, S. H., Lovinger, D. M., Ohno-Shosaku, T., & Watanabe, M. (2015). Weeding out bad waves: towards selective cannabinoid circuit control in epilepsy. *Nature reviews. Neuroscience, 16*(5), 264–277. https://doi.org/10.1038/nrn3937

Soliman, E., & Van Dross, R. (2016). Anandamide-induced endoplasmic reticulum stress and apoptosis are mediated by oxidative stress in non-melanoma skin cancer: Receptor-independent endocannabinoid signaling. *Molecular carcinogenesis, 55*(11), 1807–1821.https://doi.org/10.1002/mc.22429

Soper, S. A., & Rasooly, A. (2016). Cancer: a global concern that demands new detection technologies. *The Analyst, 141*(2), 367–370. https://doi.org/10.1039/c5an90101d

Sparling, P. B., Giuffrida, A., Piomelli, D., Rosskopf, L., & Dietrich, A. (2003). Exercise activates the endocannabinoid system. *Neuroreport, 14*(17), 2209–2211. https://doi.org/10.1097/00001756-200312020-00015

Spisni, E., Imbesi, V., Giovanardi, E., Petrocelli, G., Alvisi, P., & Valerii, M. C. (2019). Differential Physiological Responses Elicited by Ancient and Heritage Wheat Cultivars Compared to Modern Ones. *Nutrients, 11*(12), 2879. https://doi.org/10.3390/nu11122879

Stamer, W. D., Golightly, S. F., Hosohata, Y., Ryan, E. P., Porter, A. C., Varga, E., Noecker, R. J., Felder, C. C., & Yamamura, H. I. (2001). Cannabinoid CB(1) receptor expression, activation and detection of endogenous ligand in trabecular meshwork and ciliary process tissues. *European journal of pharmacology, 431*(3), 277–286. https://doi.org/10.1016/s0014-2999(01)01438-8

Starowicz, K., Makuch, W., Osikowicz, M., Piscitelli, F., Petrosino, S., Di Marzo, V., & Przewlocka, B. (2012). Spinal anandamide produces analgesia in neuropathic rats: possible CB(1)- and TRPV1- mediated mechanisms. *Neuropharmacology, 62*(4), 1746–1755. https://doi.org/10.1016/j.neuropharm.2011.11.021

Steffens, S., Veillard, N. R., Arnaud, C., Pelli, G., Burger, F., Staub, C., Karsak, M., Zimmer, A., Frossard, J. L., & Mach, F. (2005). Low dose oral cannabinoid therapy reduces progression of atherosclerosis in mice. *Nature, 434*(7034), 782–786. https://doi.org/10.1038/nature03389

Steptoe, A., Gibson, E. L., Vuononvirta, R., Williams, E. D., Hamer, M., Rycroft, J. A., Erusalimsky, J. D., & Wardle, J. (2007). The effects of tea on psychophysiological stress responsivity and post-stress recovery: a randomised double-blind trial. *Psychopharmacology, 190*(1), 81–89. https://doi.org/10.1007/s00213-006-0573-2

Storozhuk M. V. (2023). Cannabidiol: potential in treatment of neurological diseases, flax as a possible natural source of cannabidiol. Frontiers in cellular neuroscience, 17, 1131653. https://doi.org/10.3389/fncel.2023.1131653

Styrczewska, M., Kulma, A., Ratajczak, K., Amarowicz, R., & Szopa, J. (2012). Cannabinoid-like anti- inflammatory compounds from flax fiber. Cellular & molecular biology letters, 17(3), 479–499. https://doi.org/10.2478/s11658-012-0023-6

Su, K. Y., Yu, C. Y., Chen, Y. W., Huang, Y. T., Chen, C. T., Wu, H. F., & Chen, Y. L. (2014). Rutin, a flavonoid and principal component of saussurea involucrata, attenuates physical fatigue in a forced swimming mouse model. International journal of medical sciences, 11(5), 528–537. https://doi.org/10.7150/ijms.8220

Supa'at, I., Zakaria, Z., Maskon, O., Aminuddin, A., & Nordin, N. A. (2013). Effects of Swedish massage therapy on blood pressure, heart rate, and inflammatory markers in hypertensive women. Evidence-based complementary and alternative medicine : eCAM, 2013, 171852.https://doi.org/10.1155/2013/171852

Suplita, R. L., 2nd, Eisenstein, S. A., Neely, M. H., Moise, A. M., & Hohmann, A. G. (2008). Cross- sensitization and cross-tolerance between exogenous cannabinoid antinociception and endocannabinoid-mediated stress-induced analgesia. Neuropharmacology, 54(1), 161–171. https://doi.org/10.1016/j.neuropharm.2007.07.006

Szuhany, K. L., Bugatti, M., & Otto, M. W. (2015). A meta-analytic review of the effects of exercise on brain-derived neurotrophic factor. Journal of psychiatric research, 60, 56–64. https://doi.org/10.1016/j.jpsychires.2014.10.003

Tadijan, A., Vlašić, I., Vlainić, J., Đikić, D., Oršolić, N., & Jazvinšćak Jembrek, M. (2022). Intracellular Molecular Targets and Signaling Pathways Involved in Antioxidative and Neuroprotective Effects of Cannabinoids in Neurodegenerative Conditions. Antioxidants (Basel, Switzerland), 11(10), 2049. https://doi.org/10.3390/antiox11102049

Takic, M., Pokimica, B., Petrovic-Oggiano, G., & Popovic, T. (2022). Effects of Dietary α-Linolenic Acid Treatment and the Efficiency of Its Conversion to Eicosapentaenoic and Docosahexaenoic Acids in Obesity and Related Diseases. Molecules (Basel, Switzerland), 27(14), 4471. https://doi.org/10.3390/molecules27144471

Tam, J., Liu, J., Mukhopadhyay, B., Cinar, R., Godlewski, G., & Kunos, G. (2011). Endocannabinoids in liver disease. Hepatology (Baltimore, Md.), 53(1), 346–355. https://doi.org/10.1002/hep.24077

Tang, T. Y., Kim, J. S., & Das, A. (2023). Role of omega-3 and omega-6 endocannabinoids in cardiopulmonary pharmacology. Advances in pharmacology (San Diego, Calif.), 97, 375–422. https://doi.org/10.1016/bs.apha.2023.02.003

Tarawneh, A. H., León, F., Ibrahim, M. A., Pettaway, S., McCurdy, C. R., & Cutler, S. J. (2014). Flavanones from Miconia prasina. Phytochemistry letters, 7, 130–132. https://doi.org/10.1016/j.phytol.2013.11.001

Taren, A. A., Creswell, J. D., & Gianaros, P. J. (2013). Dispositional mindfulness co-varies with smaller amygdala and caudate volumes in community adults. PloS one, 8(5), e64574. https://doi.org/10.1371/journal.pone.0064574

Tashkin D. P. (2013). Effects of marijuana smoking on the lung. Annals of the American Thoracic Society, 10(3), 239–247. https://doi.org/10.1513/AnnalsATS.201212-127FR

Taylor, A. G., Snyder, A. E., Anderson, J. G., Brown, C. J., Densmore, J. J., & Bourguignon, C. (2014). Gentle Massage Improves Disease- and Treatment-Related Symptoms in Patients with Acute Myelogenous Leukemia. Journal of clinical trials, 4, 1000161. https://doi.org/10.4172/2167-0870.1000161

Teixeira-Clerc, F., Julien, B., Grenard, P., Tran Van Nhieu, J., Deveaux, V., Li, L., Serriere-Lanneau, V., Ledent, C., Mallat, A., & Lotersztajn, S. (2006). CB1 cannabinoid receptor antagonism: a new strategy for the treatment of liver fibrosis. Nature medicine, 12(6), 671–676. https://doi.org/10.1038/nm1421

Thaker, G. K., & Carpenter, W. T., Jr (2001). Advances in schizophrenia. Nature medicine, 7(6), 667–671. https://doi.org/10.1038/89040

Tharmalingam, J., Gangadaran, P., Rajendran, R. L., & Ahn, B. C. (2024). Impact of Alcohol on Inflammation, Immunity, Infections, and Extracellular Vesicles in Pathogenesis. Cureus, 16(3), e56923. https://doi.org/10.7759/cureus.56923

Thors, L., Belghiti, M., & Fowler, C. J. (2008). Inhibition of fatty acid amide hydrolase by kaempferol and related naturally occurring flavonoids. *British journal of pharmacology, 155*(2), 244–252. https://doi.org/10.1038/bjp.2008.237

Thors, L., Burston, J. J., Alter, B. J., McKinney, M. K., Cravatt, B. F., Ross, R. A., Pertwee, R. G., Gereau, R. W., 4th, Wiley, J. L., & Fowler, C. J. (2010). Biochanin A, a naturally occurring inhibitor of fatty acid amide hydrolase. *British journal of pharmacology, 160*(3), 549–560. https://doi.org/10.1111/j.1476-5381.2010.00716.x

Toguri, J. T., Lehmann, C., Laprairie, R. B., Szczesniak, A. M., Zhou, J., Denovan-Wright, E. M., & Kelly, M. E. (2014). Anti-inflammatory effects of cannabinoid CB(2) receptor activation in endotoxin- induced uveitis. *British journal of pharmacology, 171*(6), 1448–1461. https://doi.org/10.1111/bph.12545

Topuz, R. D., Gündüz, Ö., Karadağ, Ç. H., & Ulugöl, A. (2020). Non-opioid Analgesics and the Endocannabinoid System. *Balkan medical journal, 37*(6), 309–315. https://doi.org/10.4274/balkanmedj.galenos.2020.2020.6.66

Tóth, A., Blumberg, P. M., & Boczán, J. (2009). Anandamide and the vanilloid receptor (TRPV1). *Vitamins and hormones, 81*, 389–419. https://doi.org/10.1016/S0083-6729(09)81015-7

Tudurí, E., Imbernon, M., Hernández-Bautista, R. J., Tojo, M., Fernø, J., Diéguez, C., & Nogueiras, R. (2017). GPR55: a new promising target for metabolism?. *Journal of molecular endocrinology, 58*(3), R191–R202. https://doi.org/10.1530/JME-16-0253

Turcotte, C., Blanchet, M. R., Laviolette, M., & Flamand, N. (2016). The CB$_2$ receptor and its role as a regulator of inflammation. *Cellular and molecular life sciences : CMLS, 73*(23), 4449–4470.https://doi.org/10.1007/s00018-016-2300-4

Tzavara, E. T., Wade, M., & Nomikos, G. G. (2003). Biphasic effects of cannabinoids on acetylcholine release in the hippocampus: site and mechanism of action. *The Journal of neuroscience : the official journal of the Society for Neuroscience, 23*(28), 9374–9384. https://doi.org/10.1523/JNEUROSCI.23-28-09374.2003

Ujike, H., & Morita, Y. (2004). New perspectives in the studies on endocannabinoid and cannabis: cannabinoid receptors and schizophrenia. *Journal of pharmacological sciences, 96*(4), 376–381. https://doi.org/10.1254/jphs.fmj04003x4

van Amsterdam, J., Brunt, T., & van den Brink, W. (2015). The adverse health effects of synthetic cannabinoids with emphasis on psychosis-like effects. *Journal of psychopharmacology (Oxford, England), 29*(3), 254–263. https://doi.org/10.1177/0269881114565142

van der Stelt, M., Mazzola, C., Esposito, G., Matias, I., Petrosino, S., De Filippis, D., Micale, V., Steardo, L., Drago, F., Iuvone, T., & Di Marzo, V. (2006). Endocannabinoids and beta-amyloid-induced neurotoxicity in vivo: effect of pharmacological elevation of endocannabinoid levels. *Cellular and molecular life sciences : CMLS, 63*(12), 1410–1424. https://doi.org/10.1007/s00018-006-6037-3

Varga, K., Lake, K., Martin, B. R., & Kunos, G. (1995). Novel antagonist implicates the CB1 cannabinoid receptor in the hypotensive action of anandamide. *European journal of pharmacology, 278*(3), 279–283. https://doi.org/10.1016/0014-2999(95)00181-j

Vasincu, A., Rusu, R. N., Ababei, D. C., Larion, M., Bild, W., Stanciu, G. D., Solcan, C., & Bild, V. (2022). Endocannabinoid Modulation in Neurodegenerative Diseases: In Pursuit of Certainty. *Biology, 11*(3), 440. https://doi.org/10.3390/biology11030440

Vaughan, C. W., & Christie, M. J. (2005). Retrograde signalling by endocannabinoids. *Handbook of experimental pharmacology*, (168), 367–383. https://doi.org/10.1007/3-540-26573-2_12

Velasco, G., Sánchez, C., & Guzmán, M. (2012). Towards the use of cannabinoids as antitumour agents. *Nature reviews. Cancer, 12*(6), 436–444. https://doi.org/10.1038/nrc3247

Velusami, C. C., Agarwal, A., & Mookambeswaran, V. (2013). Effect of Nelumbo nucifera Petal Extracts on Lipase, Adipogenesis, Adipolysis, and Central Receptors of Obesity. *Evidence-based complementary and alternative medicine : eCAM, 2013*, 145925. https://doi.org/10.1155/2013/145925

Venkatakrishna, K., Sundeep, K., Sudeep, H. V., Gouthamchandra, K., & Shyamprasad, K. (2022). Viphyllin™, a Standardized Black Pepper Seed Extract Exerts Antinociceptive Effects in Murine Pain Models via Activation of Cannabinoid Receptor CB2, Peroxisome Proliferator-Activated Receptor-Alpha and TRPV1 Ion Channels. *Journal of pain research*, 15, 355–366. https://doi.org/10.2147/JPR.S351513

Verberne, L., Bach-Faig, A., Buckland, G., & Serra-Majem, L. (2010). Association between the Mediterranean diet and cancer risk: a review of observational studies. *Nutrition and cancer*, 62(7), 860–870. https://doi.org/10.1080/01635581.2010.509834

Vighi, G., Marcucci, F., Sensi, L., Di Cara, G., & Frati, F. (2008). Allergy and the gastrointestinal system. *Clinical and experimental immunology*, 153 Suppl 1(Suppl 1), 3–6. https://doi.org/10.1111/j.1365-2249.2008.03713.x

Vinod, K. Y., Yalamanchili, R., Xie, S., Cooper, T. B., & Hungund, B. L. (2006). Effect of chronic ethanol exposure and its withdrawal on the endocannabinoid system. *Neurochemistry international*, 49(6), 619–625. https://doi.org/10.1016/j.neuint.2006.05.002

Wade, D. T., Robson, P., House, H., Makela, P., & Aram, J. (2003). A preliminary controlled study to determine whether whole-plant cannabis extracts can improve intractable neurogenic symptoms. *Clinical rehabilitation*, 17(1), 21–29. https://doi.org/10.1191/0269215503cr581oa

Waksman, Y., Olson, J. M., Carlisle, S. J., & Cabral, G. A. (1999). The central cannabinoid receptor (CB1) mediates inhibition of nitric oxide production by rat microglial cells. *The Journal of pharmacology and experimental therapeutics*, 288(3), 1357–1366.

Waldman, M., Hochhauser, E., Fishbein, M., Aravot, D., Shainberg, A., & Sarne, Y. (2013). An ultra-low dose of tetrahydrocannabinol provides cardioprotection. *Biochemical pharmacology*, 85(11), 1626–1633. https://doi.org/10.1016/j.bcp.2013.03.014

Wallace, M. J., Martin, B. R., & DeLorenzo, R. J. (2002). Evidence for a physiological role of endocannabinoids in the modulation of seizure threshold and severity. *European journal of pharmacology*, 452(3), 295–301. https://doi.org/10.1016/s0014-2999(02)02331-2

Walsh, S. K., Hepburn, C. Y., Kane, K. A., & Wainwright, C. L. (2010). Acute administration of cannabidiol in vivo suppresses ischaemia-induced cardiac arrhythmias and reduces infarct size when given at reperfusion. *British journal of pharmacology*, 160(5), 1234–1242. https://doi.org/10.1111/j.1476-5381.2010.00755.x

Walther, S., Mahlberg, R., Eichmann, U., & Kunz, D. (2006). Delta-9-tetrahydrocannabinol for nighttime agitation in severe dementia. *Psychopharmacology*, 185(4), 524–528. https://doi.org/10.1007/s00213-006-0343-1

Wang, Q., Li, X., Chen, Y., Wang, F., Yang, Q., Chen, S., Min, Y., Li, X., & Xiong, L. (2011). Activation of epsilon protein kinase C-mediated anti-apoptosis is involved in rapid tolerance induced by electroacupuncture pretreatment through cannabinoid receptor type 1. *Stroke*, 42(2), 389–396. https://doi.org/10.1161/STROKEAHA.110.597336

Watson, J. E., Kim, J. S., & Das, A. (2019). Emerging class of omega-3 fatty acid endocannabinoids & their derivatives. *Prostaglandins & other lipid mediators*, 143, 106337. https://doi.org/10.1016/j.prostaglandins.2019.106337

Weiss, L., Zeira, M., Reich, S., Slavin, S., Raz, I., Mechoulam, R., & Gallily, R. (2008). Cannabidiol arrests onset of autoimmune diabetes in NOD mice. *Neuropharmacology*, 54(1), 244–249. https://doi.org/10.1016/j.neuropharm.2007.06.029

White, J. P., Urban, L., & Nagy, I. (2011). TRPV1 function in health and disease. *Current pharmaceutical biotechnology*, 12(1), 130–144. https://doi.org/10.2174/138920111793937844

Wilson, J. B., Epstein, M., Lopez, B., Brown, A. K., Lutfy, K., & Friedman, T. C. (2023). The role of Neurochemicals, Stress Hormones and Immune System in the Positive Feedback Loops between Diabetes, Obesity and Depression. *Frontiers in endocrinology*, 14, 1224612. https://doi.org/10.3389/fendo.2023.1224612

Woelkart, K., Xu, W., Pei, Y., Makriyannis, A., Picone, R. P., & Bauer, R. (2005). The endocannabinoid system as a target for alkamides from Echinacea angustifolia roots. *Planta medica*, 71(8), 701–705. https://doi.org/10.1055/s-2005-871290

Wolf, S. A., Bick-Sander, A., Fabel, K., Leal-Galicia, P., Tauber, S., Ramirez-Rodriguez, G., Müller, A., Melnik, A., Waltinger, T. P., Ullrich, O., & Kempermann, G. (2010). Cannabinoid receptor CB1 mediates baseline and activity-induced survival of new neurons in adult hippocampal neurogenesis. *Cell communication and signaling : CCS*, 8, 12. https://doi.org/10.1186/1478-811X-8-12

Wong, B. S., Camilleri, M., Busciglio, I., Carlson, P., Szarka, L. A., Burton, D., & Zinsmeister, A. R. (2011). Pharmacogenetic trial of a cannabinoid agonist shows reduced fasting colonic motility in patients with nonconstipated irritable bowel syndrome. *Gastroenterology*, 141(5), 1638– 47.e477. https://doi.org/10.1053/j.gastro.2011.07.036

Wright, K. L., Duncan, M., & Sharkey, K. A. (2008). Cannabinoid CB2 receptors in the gastrointestinal tract: a regulatory system in states of inflammation. *British journal of pharmacology*, 153(2), 263–270. https://doi.org/10.1038/sj.bjp.0707486

Xie, C., Liu, G., Liu, J., Huang, Z., Wang, F., Lei, X., Wu, X., Huang, S., Zhong, D., & Xu, X. (2012). Anti- proliferative effects of anandamide in human hepatocellular carcinoma cells. *Oncology letters*, 4(3), 403–407. https://doi.org/10.3892/ol.2012.751

Xu, X., Liu, Y., Huang, S., Liu, G., Xie, C., Zhou, J., Fan, W., Li, Q., Wang, Q., Zhong, D., & Miao, X. (2006). Overexpression of cannabinoid receptors CB1 and CB2 correlates with improved prognosis of patients with hepatocellular carcinoma. *Cancer genetics and cytogenetics*, 171(1), 31–38. https://doi.org/10.1016/j.cancergencyto.2006.06.014

Yang, L., Li, Y., Ren, J., Zhu, C., Fu, J., Lin, D., & Qiu, Y. (2014). Celastrol attenuates inflammatory and neuropathic pain mediated by cannabinoid receptor type 2. *International journal of molecular sciences*, 15(8), 13637–13648. https://doi.org/10.3390/ijms150813637

Yuliana, N. D., Iqbal, M., Jahangir, M., Wijaya, C. H., Korthout, H., Kottenhage, M., Kim, H. K., & Verpoorte, R. (2011). Screening of selected Asian spices for anti obesity-related bioactivities. *Food chemistry*, 126(4), 1724–1729. https://doi.org/10.1016/j.foodchem.2010.12.066

Zada, W., VanRyzin, J. W., Perez-Pouchoulen, M., Baglot, S. L., Hill, M. N., Abbas, G., Clark, S. M., Rashid, U., McCarthy, M. M., & Mannan, A. (2022). Fatty acid amide hydrolase inhibition and N- arachidonoylethanolamine modulation by isoflavonoids: A novel target for upcoming antidepressants. *Pharmacology research & perspectives*, 10(5), e00999. https://doi.org/10.1002/prp2.999

Zarei, S., Carr, K., Reiley, L., Diaz, K., Guerra, O., Altamirano, P. F., Pagani, W., Lodin, D., Orozco, G., & Chinea, A. (2015). A comprehensive review of amyotrophic lateral sclerosis. *Surgical neurology international*, 6, 171. https://doi.org/10.4103/2152-7806.169561

Zhang, J., Chen, L., Su, T., Cao, F., Meng, X., Pei, L., Shi, J., Pan, H. L., & Li, M. (2010). Electroacupuncture increases CB2 receptor expression on keratinocytes and infiltrating inflammatory cells in inflamed skin tissues of rats. *The journal of pain*, 11(12), 1250–1258. https://doi.org/10.1016/j.jpain.2010.02.013

Zhang, Z., Guo, Y., Zhang, S., Zhang, Y., Wang, Y., Ni, W., Kong, D., Chen, W., & Zheng, S. (2013). Curcumin modulates cannabinoid receptors in liver fibrosis in vivo and inhibits extracellular matrix expression in hepatic stellate cells by suppressing cannabinoid receptor type-1 in vitro. *European journal of pharmacology*, 721(1-3), 133–140. https://doi.org/10.1016/j.ejphar.2013.09.042

Zhuang, S., Kittler, J., Grigorenko, E. V., Kirby, M. T., Sim, L. J., Hampson, R. E., Childers, S. R., & Deadwyler, S. A. (1998). Effects of long-term exposure to delta9-THC on expression of cannabinoid receptor (CB1) mRNA in different rat brain regions. *Brain research. Molecular brain research*, 62(2), 141–149. https://doi.org/10.1016/s0169-328x(98)00232-0

Zou, S., & Kumar, U. (2018). Cannabinoid Receptors and the Endocannabinoid System: Signaling and Function in the Central Nervous System. *International journal of molecular sciences*, 19(3), 833. https://doi.org/10.3390/ijms19030833

www.ingramcontent.com/pod-product-compliance
Lightning Source LLC
Chambersburg PA
CBHW050502290526
45786CB00006B/2403